Cutaneous Neural Neoplasms

Current Clinical Pathology

ANTONIO GIORDANO, MD, PHD

SERIES EDITOR

For other titles published in this series, go to
www.springer.com/series/7632

Zsolt Argenyi • Chris H. Jokinen

Cutaneous Neural Neoplasms

A Practical Guide

Humana Press

Zsolt Argenyi, M.D.
Professor of Pathology and Dermatology
Director of Dermatopathology Division
1959 NE Pacific St.
98195-6100 Seattle Washington
USA
zsolt@u.washington.edu

Chris H. Jokinen, M.D.
Essentia Health, Duluth Clinic
Department of Pathology
407 East Third Street
55811 Duluth Minnesota
USA
cjokinen@smdc.org

ISBN 978-1-4939-5769-9 ISBN 978-1-60327-582-8 (eBook)
DOI 10.1007/978-1-60327-582-8
Springer New York Dordrecht Heidelberg London

Softcover re-print of the Hardcover 1st edition 2011

Printed on acid-free paper

Humana Press is part of Springer Science+Business Media (www.springer.com)

This work is dedicated to the memory of my father.

—ZA

This work is dedicated to Shawna for your support, patience and strength.

—CHJ

Preface

Cutaneous neuropathology seems a small and esoteric field within the extensive domain of dermatopathology. Paradoxically, tumors of this category include some of the most vexing problems that dermatopathologists encounter in their daily practice. Since peripheral neural tumors are soft tissue tumors, they are studied and diagnosed by general pathologists or by soft tissue specialists. However, many neural tumors that occur in the skin or in superficial soft tissues are first seen by dermatologists or by dermatopathologists, who may not be familiar with the fine details of relevant neuropathology. Because of this division of diagnostic histopathology, cutaneous neuropathology became somewhat of a "no man's land." Present monograph intends to fill this gap in diagnostic dermatopathology. It is a practical guide with abundant illustrations of variants of common cutaneous neural neoplasms. Like any field of medicine, cutaneous neuropathology is ever evolving; therefore, changes in nomenclature and classification can be expected. For practical reasons we have used the current terminology and accepted classification with the understanding that the definition of some entities may change.

Regardless of the most recent concepts of pathogenesis, every skin lesion should be classified for the ultimate purpose of diagnostic pathology, namely for better treatment of the patient. In this book the discussion of entities is based on the knowledge of normal histology and familiarity with histogenetic considerations. Naturally, the evidence-based diagnosis should be supported by consistent use of ancillary diagnostic tools.

The reader will find in this book ample drawings, 3D schematic illustrations, flowcharts, and tables beside traditional microphotographs. Numerous immunohistochemical illustrations should assist to solve the diagnostic problem at hand. The key clinical and histological findings have been concisely described, but the main emphasis is on helpful illustrations. The reader is encouraged to follow a conceptual approach to these tumors, i.e., first to understand the definition of an entity and then to correlate the histologic findings with the postulated histogenesis. Although many of these histogenetic ideas remain putative, they can guide in the analysis of characteristic morphologic appearance and help in the formulation of diagnostic criteria.

Finally, the reader may be interested in the history of this book. The idea was conceived about 20 years ago when the senior author (ZA) became interested in cutaneous neural tumors and recognized the lack of a pertinent monograph. This intention was strongly encouraged and supported by Bernard Ackerman, a prominent leader and contributor in the field of dermatopathology. Almost simultaneously, the senior author also had the honor to learn from Richard Reed, a general pathologist with vast experience in dermatopathology and a pioneer in cutaneous neuropathology, and thanks to his generosity, the senior author had the opportunity to collaborate with him on several book chapters. Although the present book was conceived in its basic form 20 years ago, due to ever-increasing professional commitments it had to remain on the back burner. Nevertheless, this field remained in the focus of the author's interest. During the past years he had reviewed in consultation an extraordinary number of unusual neural tumors, which greatly contributed to his understanding. As a result, this book has benefited from the accumulated knowledge during this period.

A major impetus for the completion of this monograph came from my former and talented dermatopathology fellow, Chris Jokinen, who expressed interest in this area. Stimulated by his enthusiasm and with his dedicated help this book has finally materialized. The authors firmly believe that the recent trend in molecular biology will further expand our understanding of cutaneous neural tumors; therefore, certain reclassification will be inevitable. While we will make efforts to include these changes in a future edition, we are confident that the reader will find the time-honored approach in this book useful in daily diagnostic work.

Seattle, WA — Zsolt Argenyi
Duluth, MN — Chris H. Jokinen

Acknowledgments

The authors express their full-hearted appreciations for the administrative support received from Eric Broeren and Virginia Lore, to Dr. Nelson Fausto, Chair, Department of Pathology, who provided the academic background for such an endeavor, to Brett Mierow for the technical assistance, and Dr. Károly Balogh, a long-time colleague and friend for his critical comments and professional support. The authors are also grateful to the staff of Humana Press/ Springer for the excellent editorial and technical assistance, which helped to bring this work into fruition.

Contents

The Peripheral Nerve and Cutaneous Neural Tumors: Introduction, Definitions, and Classification

1

Keywords
Classifications • Terminology • Normal histology • Histogenesis • Ultrastructure • Normal peripheral nerve

Peripheral nerves, brain, and spinal cord comprise the neural organ system, which is traditionally divided by its components into the peripheral nervous system and central nervous system. Cutaneous peripheral nerves are responsible for the transmission of sensory information, motor function, and control of multiple functions vital to preservation of the integument and survival of the human. Among these are sensory of the external environment through touch and pressure, and temperature regulation by control over erector pili muscle, eccrine duct secretion for sweating, and constriction or dilation of blood vessels for conservation or release of heat. The peripheral component of the neural organ system includes nerve fibers, nerve fascicles, and various sensory receptors.

The basic unit of the peripheral nerve is the *nerve fiber*, which is composed of an axon and Schwann cells (Fig. 1.1). *Axons* are long cytoplasmic extensions of a neuron whose cell body is located either in the ganglionic chain or central nervous system. Ascending sensory nerve axons attach to cell bodies located in the dorsal root ganglia. Motor axons descend from cell bodies in the ventral horn of the spinal cord, motor nuclei in the brain stem, or sympathetic and parasympathetic ganglia. Axons contain microfilaments, specialized intermediate filaments (neural filaments) and microtubules. *Schwann cells* are specialized neurosustentacular cells that provide support for axons and contribute to the propagation of transmitted stimuli. Schwann cells are encased by a continuous basal lamina and also contain intermediate filaments.

Axons can be myelinated or unmyelinated. Myelinated axons are sheathed by multiple rotations of Schwann cell cytoplasmic membranes, resulting in increased velocity of neural transmissions (action potentials). Unmyelinated axons are also bounded by the cytoplasm of the Schwann cells but without the multiple rotations found in myelinated forms. Axons end directly in the epidermis or on cells of the cutaneous adnexal structures or smooth muscle. Sensory axons are connected to specialized mechanoreceptors, such as the corpuscles of Pacini, Ruffini, or Meissner; hair follicle receptors; and Merkel cells.

A *nerve fascicle* is a bundled collection of multiple nerve fibers, which constitutes the tissue-based component of the peripheral nerve upon entering the skin. Nerve fascicles are usually the most evident neural structures at the light microscopic level (Figs. 1.2a, b, 1.3, and 1.4). Characteristic examples of the most common mechanoreceptors are illustrated in Figs. 1.5–1.7.

The space between individual nerve fibers within the fascicle is called *endoneurium*. The endoneurium is composed of fibrocytes/fibroblasts and mast cells embedded in a collagenous stroma with abundant capillaries.

Z. Argenyi and C.H. Jokinen (eds.), *Cutaneous Neural Neoplasms*, Current Clinical Pathology,
DOI 10.1007/978-1-60327-582-8_1, © Springer Science+Business Media, LLC 2011

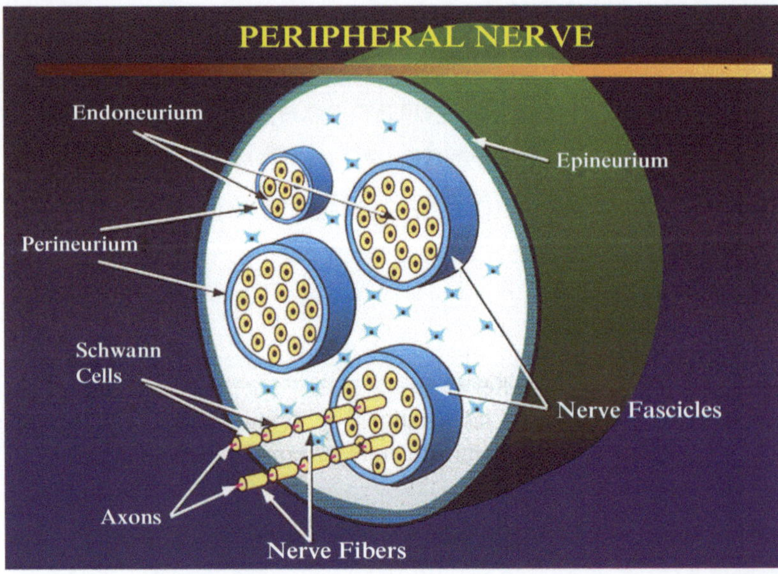

Fig. 1.1 Peripheral nerve: nerve fibers are composed of axons, surrounding Schwann cells, and supportive stromal cells. Individual nerve fascicles are encompassed by perineurium. The nerve fascicles are in turn surrounded by stroma, which is held together by epineurium forming the nerve (artwork by ZA)

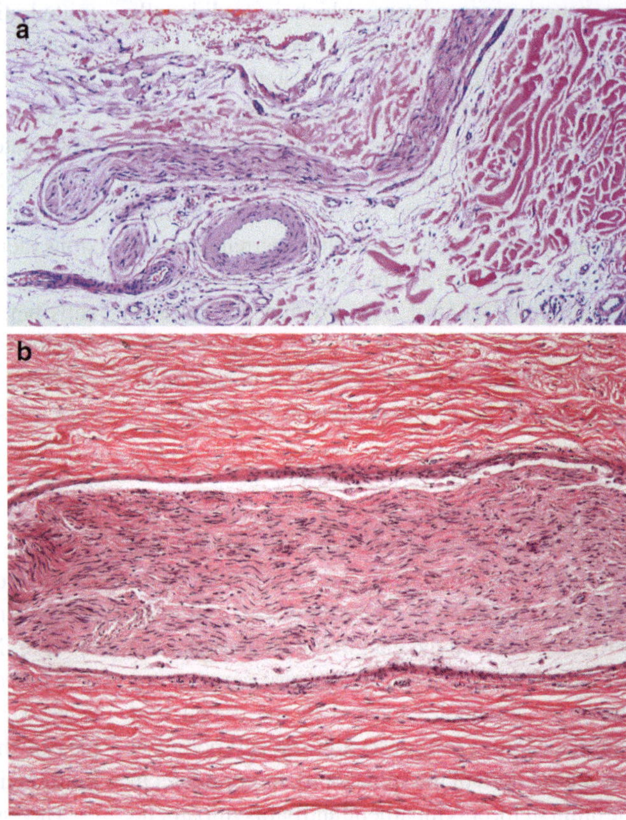

Fig. 1.2 Peripheral nerve fascicle: longitudinal sections of nerve fascicles in the subcutis (**a**) and soft tissue adjacent to a traumatic neuroma (**b**). The fascicles are composed of closely aligned Schwann cells with elongated slender nuclei. The entire fascicle is surrounded by perineurium

Collagen fibrils of the endoneurium are often partially surrounded by Schwann cell cytoplasmic processes. This suggests that Schwann cells, in part, produce collagen fibrils. Immunohistochemical evidence of type IV collagen in Schwann cells (Chap. 2) and Schwann cell neoplasms further supports this role.

The nerve fibers in a fascicle are held together by a sheath of *perineurium*, a layer that is continuous with the pia–arachnoid lining of the central

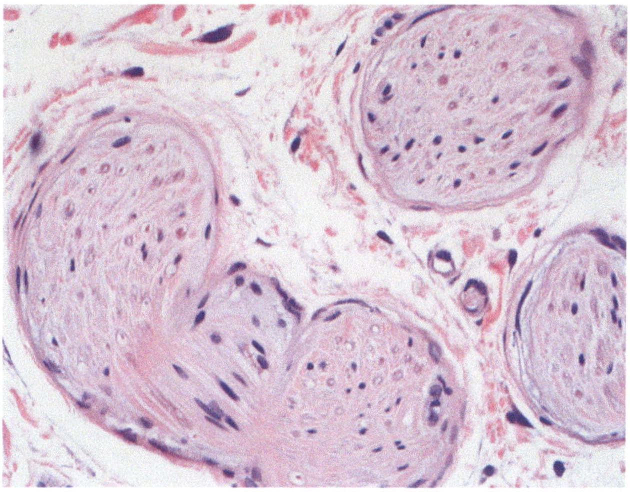

Fig. 1.3 Peripheral nerve fascicles in cross section highlight the dot-like appearance of Schwann cell nuclei when cut perpendicular to the plane of direction. Axons are difficult to visualize but are located by the clear space surrounding them. Individual neural filaments can be viewed with immunohistochemistry. Perineurial cells have slender nuclei with elongated cytoplasmic processes

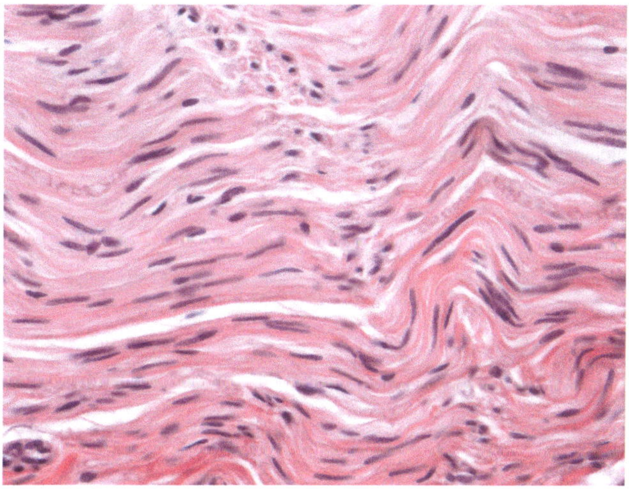

Fig. 1.4 Schwann cells have slender elongated nuclei with one tapered and one blunt end. The nuclear chromatin is fine and uniform. The cells have eosinophilic elongated cytoplasmic processes

nervous system (Fig. 1.1). Perineurium is composed of perineurial cells and collagen. Perineurial cells have flattened thin nuclei, and elongated, slender cytoplasmic extensions. Ultrastructurally, they have tight intercellular junctions, a discontinuous basal lamina and pinocytotic vesicles. Multiple layers of perineurial cells are present around each fascicle. The thickness is variable but may be up to ten cells. This barrier is responsible for separation of the nerve from the adjacent interstitium and its cellular and fluidic components.

Epineurium is an additional supportive sheath that surrounds collections of perineurium-bound nerve fascicles known as the *peripheral nerve* (Fig. 1.1). Epineurium surrounds the peripheral nerve as it exists within its own organ system but is not present within the skin. The epineurium is made up of fibrocytes, collagen, elastin fibers, and blood vessels. The collagen fibrils are large compared to those of the perineurium and endoneurium and are believed to play the major role in structural support.

In this work, the term *tumors* will be used to refer to any number of neoplasms, hamartomas, or heterotopias of neural lineage found in the skin. "Tumor" by definition is a mass. Although often used synonymously with "neoplasm," any number of neoplastic or nonneoplastic proliferations of the peripheral nerve may form a tumor.

Neoplasms are proliferations presumably derived from a single abnormal progenitor cell with aberrant regulation of cell division or growth

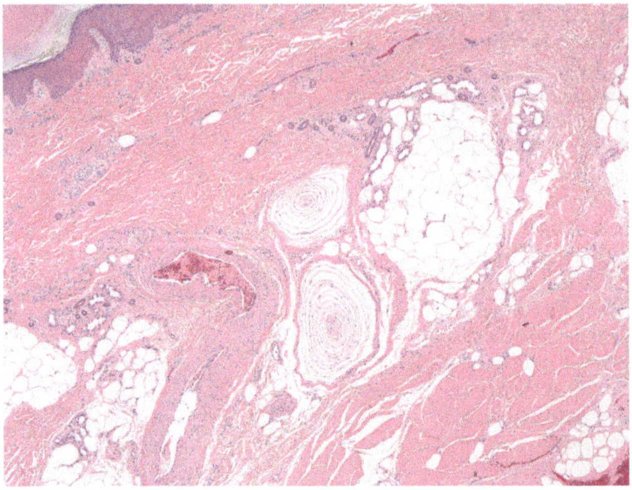

Fig. 1.5 Pacinian corpuscles are located in the reticular dermis of subcutis in acral skin. They are often located near medium-sized muscular blood vessels

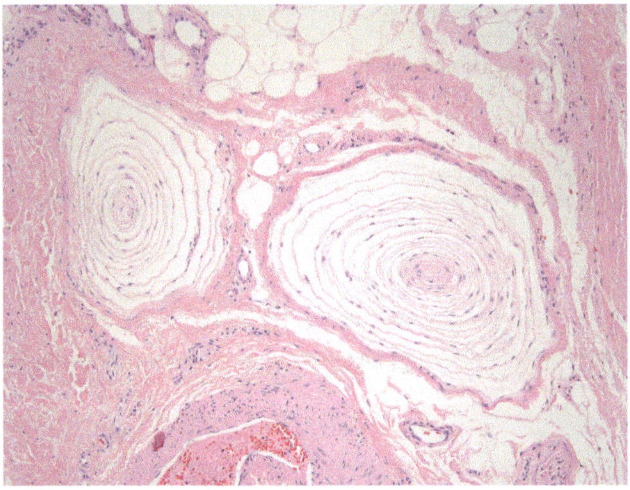

Fig. 1.6 Pacinian corpuscles are composed of a central nerve fiber surrounded by concentric layers of cells with elongated cytoplasmic processes

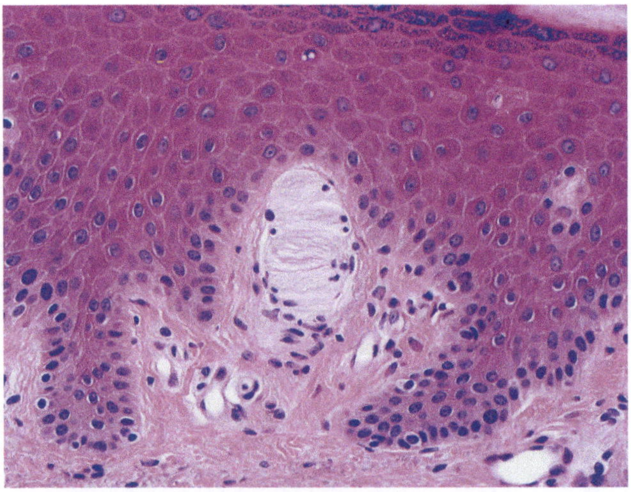

Fig. 1.7 Meissner corpuscles are touch receptors located in the dermal papillae of acral skin. They appear as round or ovoid bodies with small peripheral nuclei and lamellar processes in the center

resulting from genetic alteration. The cell of origin for cutaneous neural neoplasms has not yet been elucidated. Furthermore, like many cutaneous and visceral neoplasms, characteristic reproducible cytogenetic or molecular anomalies are not yet known for many of these lesions. As a general rule, however, cutaneous neoplasms that derive from or differentiate toward the peripheral nerve often attempt to reconstitute some architectural features of the normal nerve. As such, classification of these neoplasms is largely based on light microscopic and immunohistochemical features that resemble those of normal microscopic anatomy. Such classification will be employed in this book to the greatest extent possible. Neoplasms are benign or malignant, distinguished only by the ability of the neoplasm to metastasize. Most cutaneous neural neoplasms are benign, and although lacking the ability for distant spread, they may result in local destruction of tissues and be clinically symptomatic. Local recurrence can occur, especially when the tumor was not completely separated from its feeding nerve. Malignant neural neoplasms of the skin are uncommon, but differ by the potential to invade lymphatic or vascular channels and spread to distal sites. Neoplasms of "low malignant potential" are malignant neoplasms that in most instances metastasize only rarely.

Hamartomas are tumors composed of cell types normally found at the site in which they arise, but which are quantitatively abnormal. While precise mechanisms that give rise to hamartomas are largely unknown, they are presumed to represent an anomaly in embryologic development, unlike neoplasms, which are genetically altered proliferations derived from a single cell. Hamartomas closely resemble the usual histologic organization of the organ in which they develop. In neural hamartomas, multiple, if not all of the elements of the respective neural tissue can be identified, while in true neoplasms, one particular cell type constitutes the bulk of the tumor. *Choristomas*, like hamartomas, are quantitatively abnormal proliferations of otherwise normal cells, but differ in that they occur at locations where the lesional cells would not normally exist.

Ectopias and *heterotopias* are otherwise normal tissues and their various cell populations are located at an abnormal site. Often this is the result

Table 1.1 Classification of cutaneous neural tumors

Cutaneous peripheral nerve sheath proliferations

- Hamartomas
  - True neuromas
    - Palisaded encapsulated neuroma/solitary circumscribed neuroma
    - Mucosal neuroma
  - Fibrolipomatous hamartoma of nerve
- Other nonneoplastic and hyperplastic proliferations
  - Traumatic neuroma
  - Reparative perineurial hyperplasia
  - Morton's neuroma (interdigital neuritis)
  - Epithelial sheath neuroma[a]
- Benign neoplasms
  - Neurofibroma[a]
  - Schwannoma
  - Granular cell tumor
  - Nerve sheath myxoma
  - Perineurioma
  - Lipoblastic nerve sheath tumor[a]
- Malignant neoplasms
  - Malignant peripheral nerve sheath tumor
  - Malignant granular cell tumor

Cutaneous proliferations of putative neural origin/differentiation

- Benign neoplasms
  - Neurothekeoma
- Malignant neoplasms
  - Primary cutaneous neuroendocrine carcinoma (Merkel cell carcinoma)
- Neurofollicular hamartoma

Cutaneous neuroblastic and ganglionic proliferations

- Benign neoplasms
  - Ganglioneuroma
  - Ganglion cell choristoma[a]
- Malignant neoplasms
  - Neuroblastoma

Cutaneous glial and meningothelial proliferations

- Heterotopias
  - Glial heterotopia (nasal glioma)
  - Meningothelial heterotopia/meningocele
- Benign neoplasms
  - Cutaneous meningioma

[a]The etiologic nature of these entities is disputed or not decidedly established. Neurofibroma is included under the neoplastic group for historical purposes

of a developmental anomaly or displacement. Most cutaneous neural ectopic or heterotopic tissues are from the central nervous system and ganglionic chain.

Classification of cutaneous neural tumors is not perfect and cannot be applied to tumors in which the neural differentiation is assumed only because of cytologic features. Generally speaking, with the aid of ancillary studies such as immunohistochemistry, the following chapters will attempt to classify these proliferations in a practical manner in order for practicing pathologists and dermatopathologists could render a specific diagnosis. Table 1.1 outlines the classification of cutaneous neural tumors employed here. In this work, we have also included several entities historically classified under the rubric of neural tumors but refutably are derived from or differentiate via a nonneural lineage. This includes primary neuroendocrine carcinoma (Merkel cell carcinoma), which may or may not be related to the normal cutaneous Merkel cell and neural crest, and the enigmatic cellular neurothekeoma whose histogenesis remains disputed.

Additional Reading

Eames RA, Gamble HJ. Schwann cell relationships in normal human cutaneous nerves. J Anat. 1970;106:417.

Gamble HJ, Eames RA. An electron microscope study of the connective tissues of human peripheral nerve. J Anat. 1964;98:655.

Reed ML, Jacoby RA. Cutaneous neuroanatomy and neuropathology. Normal nerves, neural-crest derivatives, and benign neural neoplasms in the skin. Am J Dermatopathol. 1983;5:335.

Sternberg S. Histology for pathologists. 2nd ed. Philadelphia, PA: Lippincott Williams & Wilkins; 1997.

Special Techniques for the Study of Cutaneous Neural Tumors

2

Keywords
Diagnostic techniques • Special stains • Histochemistry • Immunohistochemistry • Electronmicroscopy • Molecular biology • Cytogenetics

A variety of histochemical and immunohistochemical methods, if employed in the appropriate context and in a suitable combination, are useful for identifying and classifying cutaneous neural tumors.

Immunoperoxidase is a commonly used method for identifying and characterizing the constituents of the peripheral nervous system. Table 2.1 provides an overview of the main immunohistochemical findings in cutaneous neural tumors. The most commonly used markers include S-100 protein (Schwann cells), neuron-specific enolase (neurons, axons), neural filaments (axons), epithelial membrane antigen (perineurial and meningothelial cells), Protein Gene Product 9.5 (PGP 9.5) (neurons, neuroendocrine cells, and others), myelin basic protein and CD57 (myelin products), glial fibrillar acidic protein (GFAP; astrocytes), collagen type IV (basal lamina of Schwann cells), chromogranin (endocrine/neuroendocrine secretory vesicle protein), and synaptophysin (neuroendocrine synaptic vesicle glycoprotein) (Figs. 2.1 and 2.2). Some of these immunohistochemical stains are nonspecific, and all reactions should be interpreted with appropriate controls and integrated with light microscopic and clinical findings.

In most modern practices, histochemical methods have fallen out of favor for routine diagnostic use. There are times, however, when these preparations may be contributory. Silver impregnations (Bodian or Bielschowsky stains) are among the traditional histochemical methods used for the demonstration of axons, which are highlighted as black fine, but sharp linear structures (Fig. 2.3). Luxol fast blue is useful to identify myelin with a tubular, finely bubbly staining reaction around cell membranes (Fig. 2.4). Trichrome stain is valuable for highlighting collagen and pentachrome stain will discern elastic fibers and muscular components (Fig. 2.5).

Electron microscopy is often a valuable ancillary tool especially in cases of undifferentiated neoplasms or when there is aberrant expression or confusing immunohistochemical reactions. Ultrastructural features of Schwann cells include abundant double layer of continuous basement membrane, which is associated with type IV collagen. Perineurial cells contain tight junctions and pinocytotic vesicles with a discontinuous external lamina. These have characteristic flattened nuclei (Figs. 2.6–2.10).

Unlike some soft tissue neoplasms arising in other organs, detection of specific genetic alterations by methods such as classical cytogenetics, FISH, or PCR is currently not widely employed for classification or diagnosis of cutaneous neural neoplasms. In part, this is because many neural

Z. Argenyi and C.H. Jokinen (eds.), *Cutaneous Neural Neoplasms*, Current Clinical Pathology,
DOI 10.1007/978-1-60327-582-8_2, © Springer Science+Business Media, LLC 2011

Table 2.1 Main immunohistochemical findings of common cutaneous neural neoplasms

Marker	S-100	Coll IV	NF	NSE	CD57 (Leu-7)	MBP	GFAP	EMA	VIM	SY	CD34	Other/ miscellaneous
Tumor												
Neurofibroma	++	++	+	++	+/–	+/–	–/+	–/+	++	–	++	
Schwannoma	+++	+++	–*	++	++	++	–/+	+capsule	++	–	+/–	
Traumatic neuroma	+++	+++	+++	++	++	++	–	++	++	–	+	
PEN	+++	+++	+++	++	++	++	–	+capsule	++	–	+	
Nerve sheath myxoma	+	+	–	–/+	+/–	–/+	–	+capsule	++	–	–/+	
Cellular neurothekeoma	–	–/+	–	–/+	–/+	–	–	–	++	–	–/+	SMSA, NC1/3
Perineurioma	–	+/–	–	–	–	–	–	+	+	–	+/–	
Granular cell tumor	++	+	–	+	+	+	–	–	++	–	–	CD68, lysozyme
MPNST	+/–	+/–	+/–	+/–	+/–	+/–	–	–	++	–	–/+	Desmin
Nasal glioma	+	+/–	+/–	+	–/+	–/+	+++	–	++	+	–	
Cutaneous meningioma	–/+	–/+	–	–/+	–	–	–	++	+	–	NA	
PNET	–/+	–	–	+	+/–	+/–	–	–	+/–	+	–**	CD99, MB-2
Ganglioneuroma	+	+	+/–	+	+/–	+/–	+/–	–	+	+	NA	
Cutaneous neuroblastoma	–/+	–	–/+	+	+/–	+/–	–	–	+/–	+	**	
PNECS	–	–	+	+	–	–	–	+	–	+/–	–	LMWK, CHG

PEN palisaded encamsulated neuroma, *MPNST* malignant peripheral nerve sheath tumor, *PNET* peripheral neuroectodermal tumor, *PNECS* neuroendocrine carcinoma of the skin, *S-100* S-100 protein, *Coll IV* collagen type IV, *NF* neural filaments, *NSE* neuron-specific enolase, *MPB* myelin basic protein, *GFAP* glial fibrillary acidic protein, *EMA* epithelial membrane antigen, *VIM* vimentin, *SY* synaptophysin, *CD99* antibody to p30/32 mic2, *MB-2* antibody to B-cell lymphoid determinations, *LMWK* low molecular weight keratin, *CHR* chromogranin, *NC1/3* melanoma marker, + weak or focal immunoreactivity, ++ fairly consistent reactivity, +++ usually strong immunoreactivity, +/– variable, immunoreactivity often present, –/+ variable, immunoreactivity often absent, – negative immunoreactivity, *NA* not applicable, * reaction only at nerve of origin, ** only a few cases studied

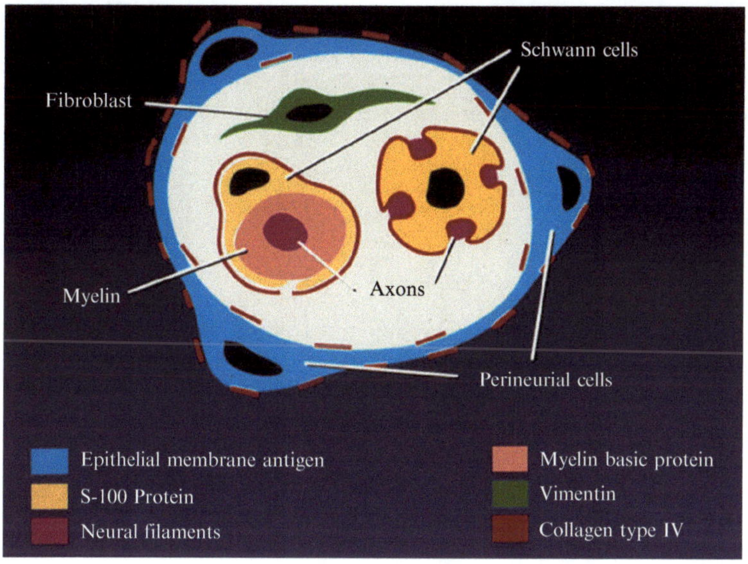

Fig. 2.1 Immunohistochemical characteristics of the peripheral nerve fascicle. In most cases, each cell population and its neoplastic counterpart can be identified by selective immunohistochemistry. Schwann cells express S-100 protein and type IV collagen and surround one axon with many rotations (myelinated) or have one or few rotations around multiple axons (unmyelinated). The former will stain with myelin basic protein. Axons are identified by neural filaments stain. Vimentin, a nonspecific marker, highlights endoneurial fibroblasts. Perineurium expresses epithelial membrane antigen and type IV collagen (artwork by ZA)

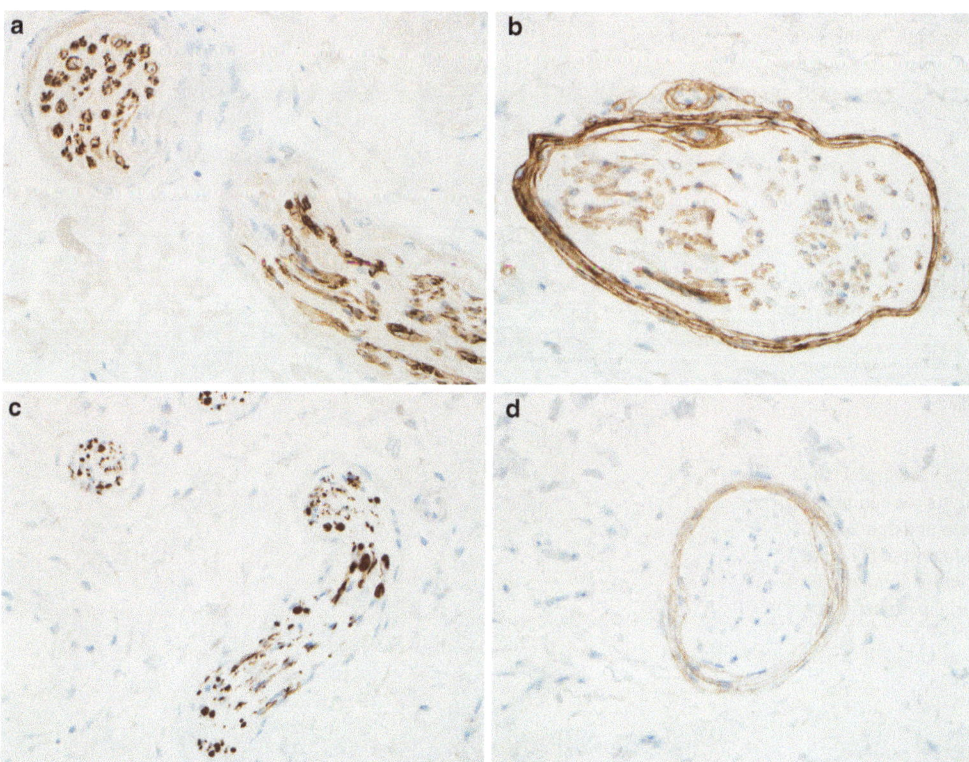

Fig. 2.2 (**a**) *S-100 protein* stains the Schwann cells. (**b**) *Type IV collagen* strongly stains the Schwann cells, perineurium, and an adjacent small vessel. (**c**) Axons are identified by a *neurofilaments* immunostain. In cross section these appear as small dots, while longitudinally appear as elongated linear structures of varying thickness. (**d**) *Epithelial membrane antigen* (*EMA*) weakly stains the perineurial cells at the periphery

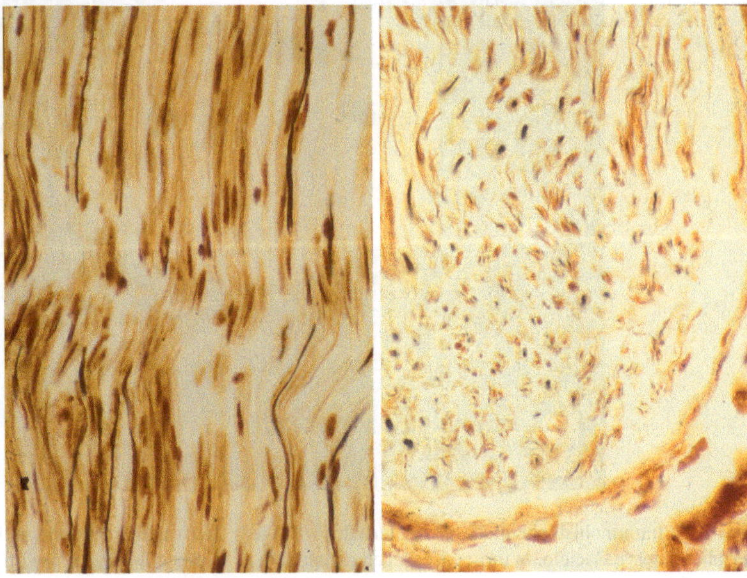

Fig. 2.3 Silver impregnation (Bielchowsky) highlights axons of a normal nerve as fine, delicate lines in longitudinal sections and as dark dot-like structures on cross sections

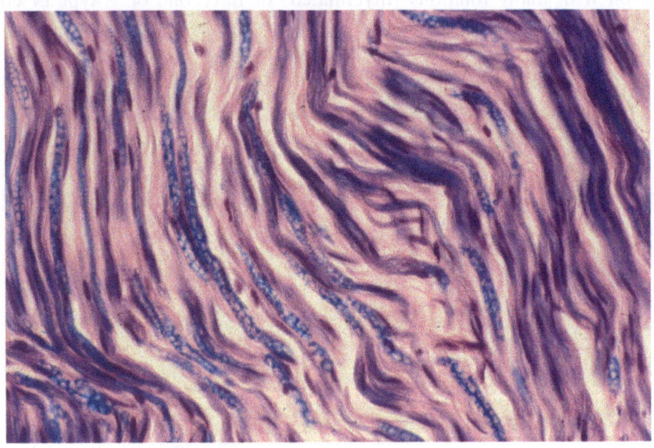

Fig. 2.4 Luxol fast blue histochemical stain highlights myelin in a larger nerve, as blue, bubbly, tubular structures along the contour of Schwann cells

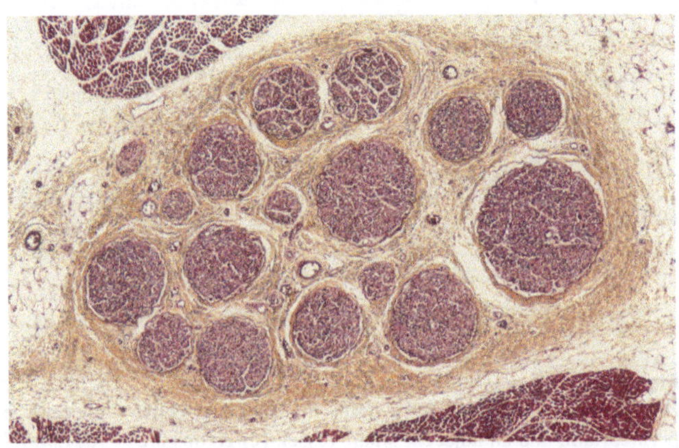

Fig. 2.5 Trichrome stain highlights the endoneurial collagen and delineates individual fascicles held together by epineurium of this large peripheral nerve

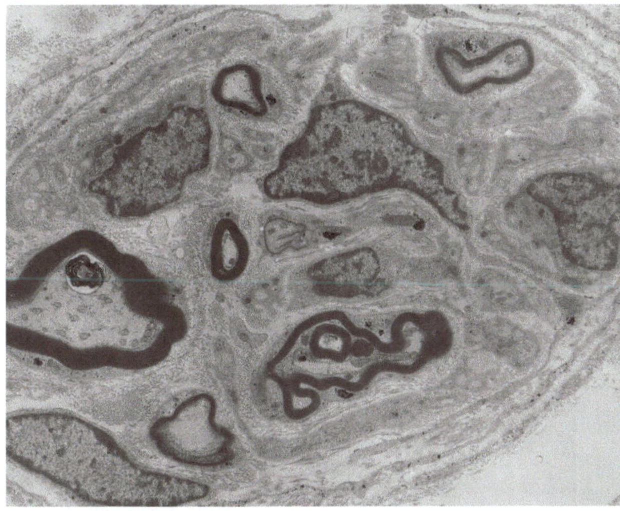

Fig. 2.6 Electronmicroscopic view of a normal cutaneous nerve, showing myelinated and unmyelinated axons, endoneurial fibroblasts, and perineurial cells (×9,000)

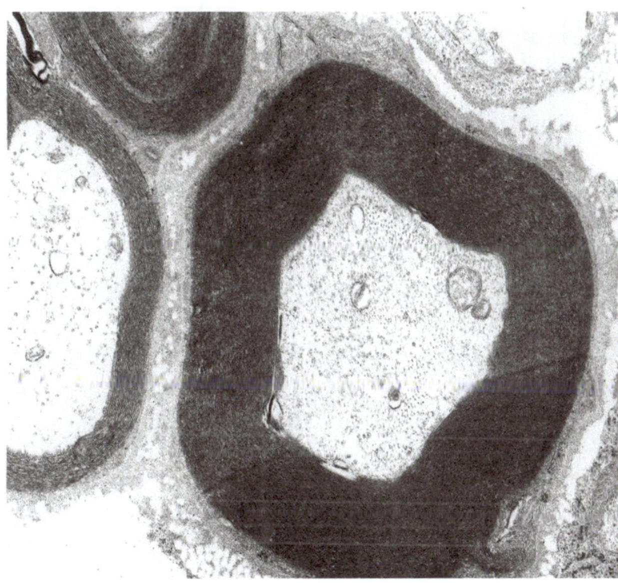

Fig. 2.7 Higher magnification of a myelinated axon shows numerous concentric layers of electron dense lamellar structures corresponding with the multiple ensheathing by a continuous basement membrane of the Schwann cells. The myelin appears black due to osmophilia. In the center there is the axon containing neurofilaments, mitochondria, and small vesicles (×38,700)

tumors are not yet known to have characteristic reproducible anomalies detectable by current methods. Also, the majority of cutaneous neural neoplasms are readily characterized by light microscopy or with the aid of immunohistochemistry. Some recurring genetic alterations are known for a subset of neural tumors. Neurofibromas arising in patients with neurofibromatosis (NF) type 1 are associated with mutations in the *neurofibromin* gene on chromosome 17. Schwannomas in patients with NF type 2 are associated with a mutation in the NF2 gene on chromosome 22q; however, this is not invariably present in sporadic forms. Perineuriomas have been associated with deletions of chromosome 22q11, translocations of chromosome 10, monosomy 10, or deletion of chromosome 13. Some meningiomas of the central nervous system have mutations of chromosome 22q as well. Many of these genetic anomalies have not been documented in cutaneous variants; however, and it remains to be determined how the classification of cutaneous neural tumors will change as additional mutations and cytogenetic anomalies are characterized.

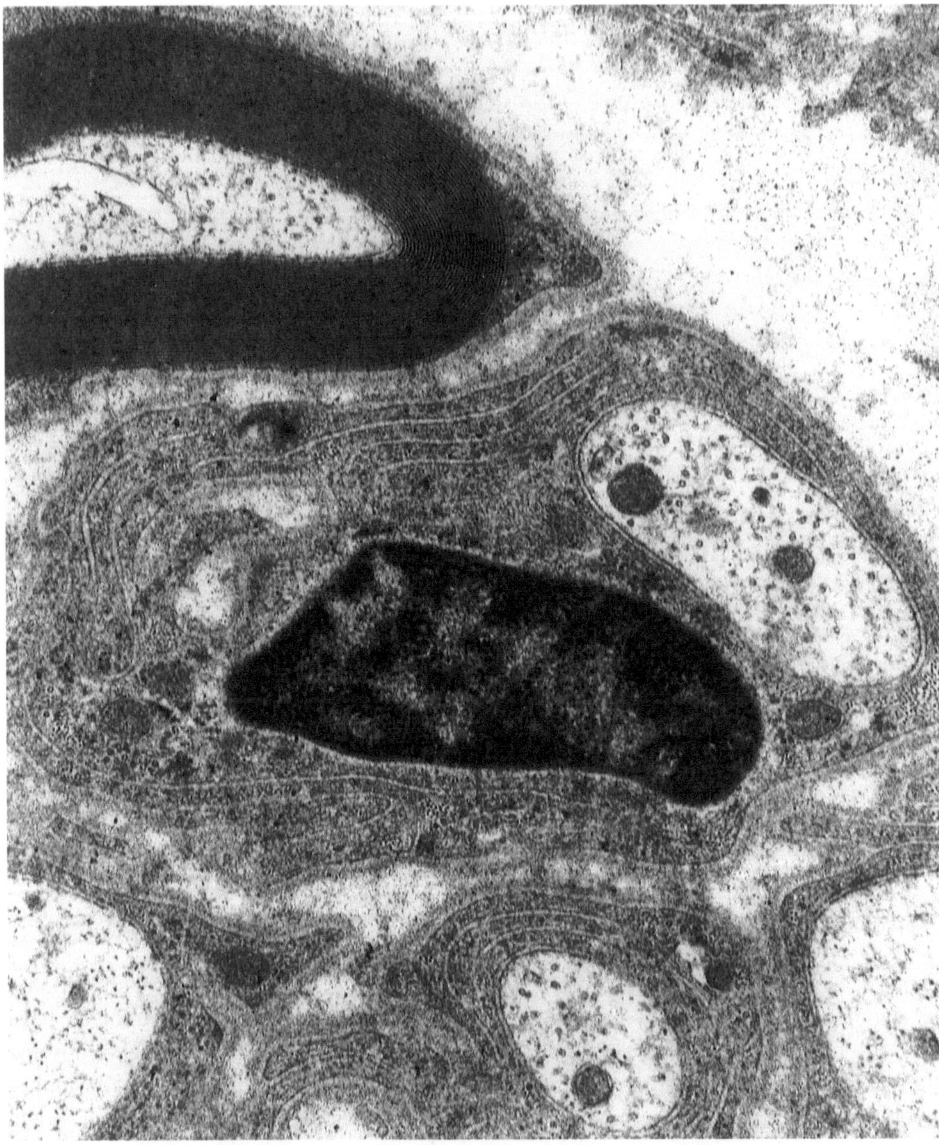

Fig. 2.8 Unmyelinated axons (*center right* and *center bottom*) are surrounded by the cytoplasmic processes of a single Schwann cell, the nucleus of which is in the center. Unlike myelinated forms, unmyelinated axons are encompassed by one or few rotations of the supporting cytoplasm. There are also microtubules within the axons. A prominent basal lamina surrounds the Schwann cells (×38,700)

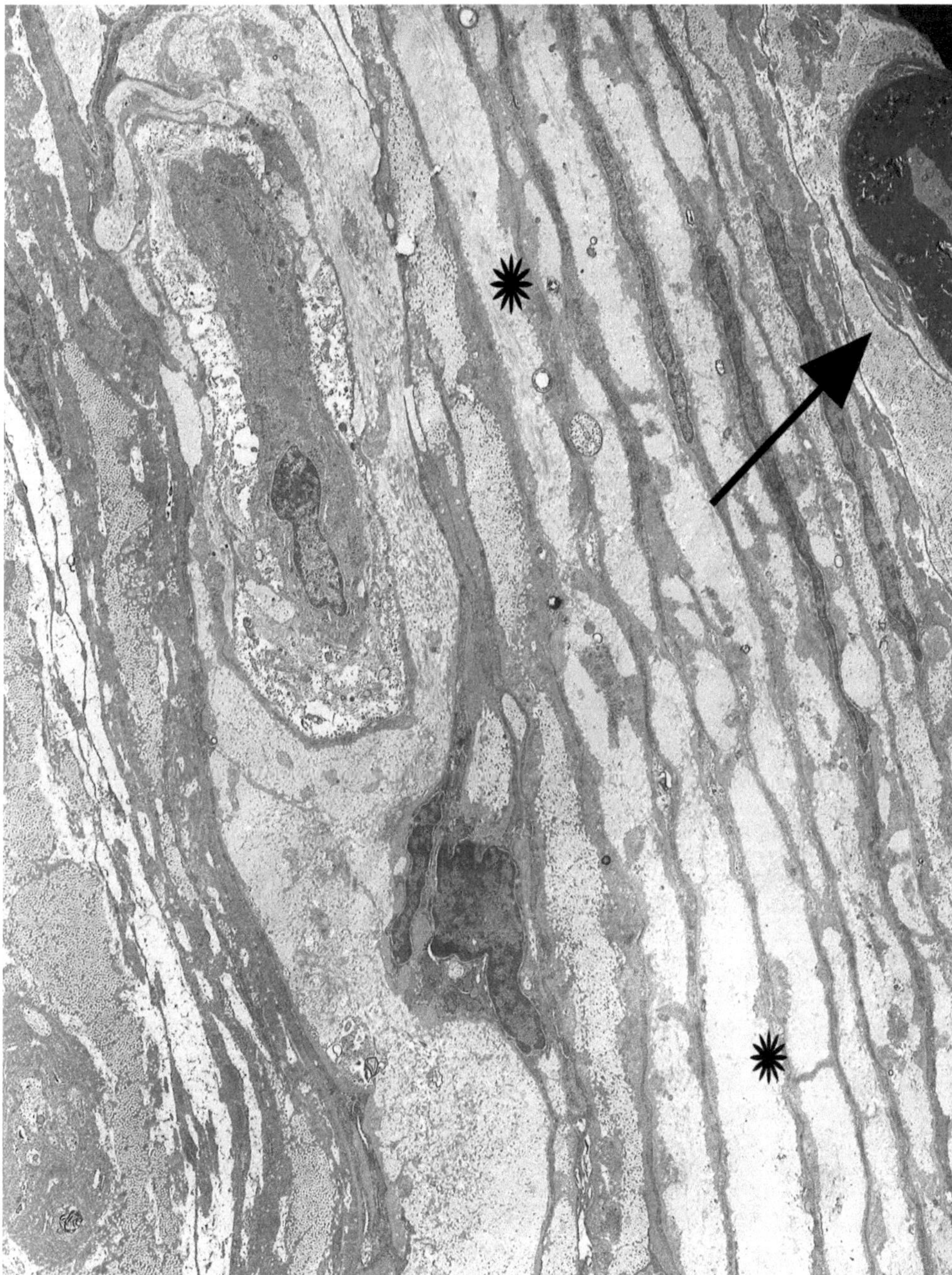

Fig. 2.9 Perineurial sheath of a normal cutaneous nerve containing several layers of elongated perineurial cells with intertwining collagen fibers. There is a myelinated fiber in the field (*arrow*) and epineurial fibroblasts (*asterisks*) outside of the perineurial cells (×5,500)

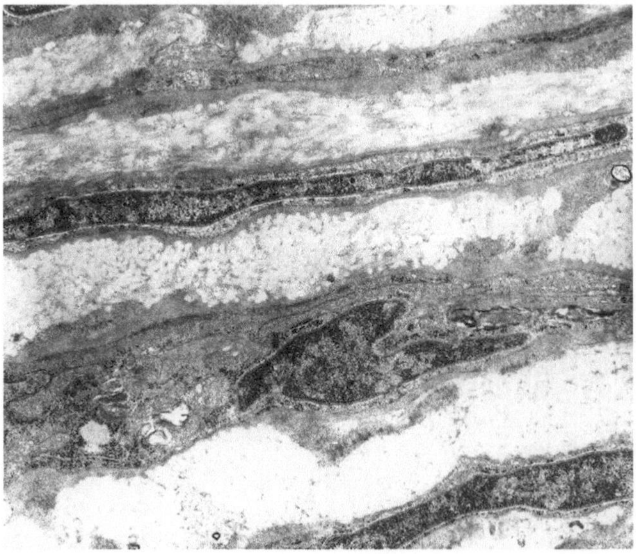

Fig. 2.10 Higher magnification of a perineurial cell shows elongated cells with a discontinuous basement membrane, and pinocytotic vesicles separated by collagen fibers (×28,750)

Additional Reading

Asthagiri AR, Parry DM, Butman JA, Kim HJ, Tsilou ET, Zhuang Z, et al. Neurofibromatosis type 2. Lancet. 2009;373:1974.

Boyd KP, Korf BR, Theos A. Neurofibromatosis type 1. J Am Acad Dermatol. 2009;61:1.

Brock JE, Perez-Atayde AR, Kozakewich HP, Richkind KE, Fletcher JA, Vargas SO. Cytogenetic aberrations in perineurioma: variation with subtype. Am J Surg Pathol. 2005;29:1164.

De Vitis LR, Tedde A, Vitelli F, Ammannati F, Mennonna P, Bigozzi U, et al. Screening for mutations in the neurofibromatosis type 2 (NF2) gene in sporadic meningiomas. Hum Genet. 1996;97:632.

Giannini C, Scheithauer BW, Jenkins RB, Erlandson RA, Perry A, Borell TJ, et al. Soft-tissue perineurioma. Evidence for an abnormality of chromosome 22, criteria for diagnosis, and review of the literature. Am J Surg Pathol. 1997;21:164.

Lasota J, Fetsch JF, Wozniak A, Wasag B, Sciot R, Miettinen M. The neurofibromatosis type 2 gene is mutated in perineurial cell tumors: a molecular genetic study of eight cases. Am J Pathol. 2001;158:1223.

Mott RT, Goodman BK, Burchette JL, Cummings TJ. Loss of chromosome 13 in a case of soft tissue perineurioma. Clin Neuropathol. 2005;24:69.

Sciot R, Dal Cin P, Hagemeijer A, De Smet L, Van Damme B, Van den Berghe H. Cutaneous sclerosing perineurioma with cryptic NF2 gene deletion. Am J Surg Pathol. 1999;23:849.

Twist EC, Ruttledge MH, Rousseau M, Sanson M, Papi L, Merel P, et al. The neurofibromatosis type 2 gene is inactivated in schwannomas. Hum Mol Genet. 1994;3:147.

Nonneoplastic and Hamartomatous Lesions of the Cutaneous Peripheral Nerve

3

Keywords
Non-neoplastic proliferations • Hamartomas • Benign tumors • Classification • Histogenesis • Diagnostic features • Differential diagnosis • Spontain and traumatic neuromas • Neuroma variants • Reparative perineurial hyperplasia

Nonneoplastic neural proliferations are among the most commonly encountered peripheral nerve sheath tumors in the skin. This chapter describes the various hamartomas (neuromas) and reparative or reactive proliferations that develop following nerve injury. In general, hamartomatous lesions of the skin constitute proliferations of each of the normal elements of the peripheral nerve fiber including Schwann cells, axons, perineurial cells, and endoneurial fibroblasts.

Palisaded Encapsulated Neuroma

Definition, Classification, and Histogenesis

Palisaded encapsulated neuroma (PEN), also known as solitary encapsulated neuroma, is a common spontaneous cutaneous neuroma. PEN is a morphologically distinctive neural hamartoma, composed of each of the elements of the normal peripheral nerve (see Fig. 3.1a, b, for line drawing). PEN is not associated with trauma, multiple endocrine neoplasia (MEN) type 2B, or an inherited predisposition to neural tumors such as neurofibromatosis.

Clinical Findings

PEN may arise at any site, but most frequently occurs on the face, often around the nose and lips. PEN is also common on the trunk and extremities. This neuroma may arise at any location, including, albeit rarely, genital and acral skin. PEN is usually a solitary white to flesh-colored firm papule. Presentation with multiple synchronous lesions is very rare. Most often PEN is clinically mistaken for a dermal nevus, adnexal neoplasm, basal cell carcinoma, or solitary neurofibroma.

Histopathology

PEN is a round or oblong nodular or polypoid proliferation that is usually well circumscribed and surrounded by a perineurial cell-rich capsule (Figs. 3.2 and 3.3). Rare variants of plexiform or interconnected nodular variants can also occur (Figs. 3.4 and 3.5). Connections between multiple nodules are usually visible. The nodules are made up of multiple closely opposed fascicles of Schwann cells and abundant axons (Figs. 3.6 and 3.7). The fascicles in most lesions are separated by prominent clefts. The clefts presumably

Z. Argenyi and C.H. Jokinen (eds.), *Cutaneous Neural Neoplasms*, Current Clinical Pathology,
DOI 10.1007/978-1-60327-582-8_3,

are an artifact of tissue processing and are among the most noticeable features at scanning magnification (Fig. 3.8). The Schwann cells may be aligned in parallel creating the appearance of nuclear palisading; however, true Verocay bodies are not present (Fig. 3.9). The typical encapsulation of PEN is often absent at the superficial aspect of the lesion near the epidermis, where the proliferation gradually blends with the dermis (Fig. 3.10). At this site, there is loss of identifiable fascicles and clefts, and the capsule usually is not discernible (or not well preserved). In some instances, this diffuse growth pattern may resemble neurofibroma and the two may be indistinguishable in a very superficial shave biopsy. The Schwann cells are spindled with fine chromatin and wavy nuclei, like that of normal nerve (Fig. 3.11). The stroma is collagenous and typically lacks myxoid change. Mitotic figures may be present, but usually are rare. The Schwann cells express S-100 protein in a diffuse and strong pattern (Fig. 3.12). A neurofilaments stain will highlight numerous axons in each fascicle, arranged parallel to the long axis of the fascicle (Fig. 3.13). Axons appear as dot-like structures when cut perpendicular to the plane of section. Epithelial membrane antigen (EMA) will stain the surrounding perineurium in a linear, continuous, or partially discontinuous pattern (Fig. 3.14).

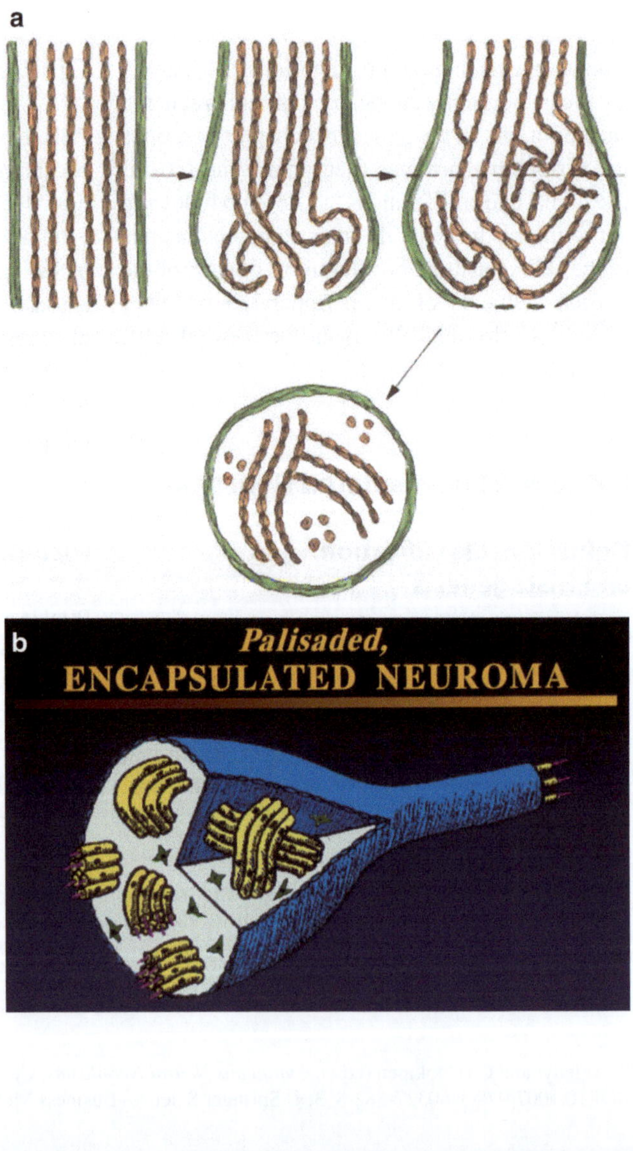

Fig. 3.1 (**a, b**) Schematic drawing of palisaded encapsulated neuroma (PEN). A normal nerve fascicle (*left*) and an expanded fascicle (*center, right*) with a proliferation of individual nerve fibers. The nerve fibers develop a tortuous growth pattern oriented along multiple planes. When cross-sectioned (*bottom*) the intersecting planes are visualized (artwork by ZA)

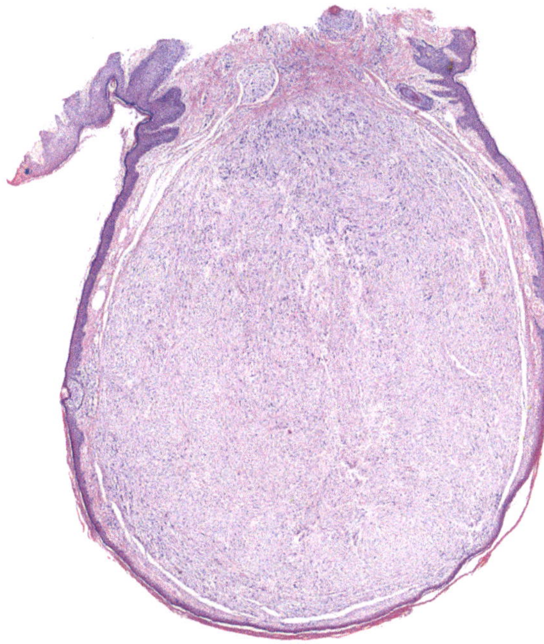

Fig. 3.2 PEN: a solitary polypoid nodule situated in the superficial dermis is the most common histopathologic presentation. Clinically, this often resembles an intradermal nevus

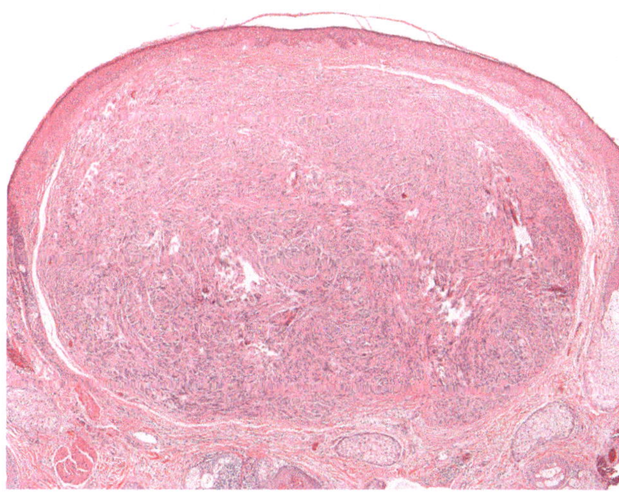

Fig. 3.3 PEN: a well-circumscribed proliferation is nearly entirely surrounded by a thin capsule of perineurium. The capsule, however, is typically absent at the superficial aspect where the lesion joins with the dermis

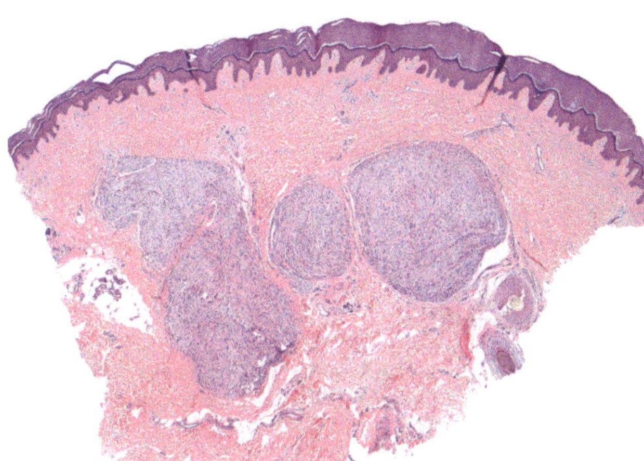

Fig. 3.4 PEN: less commonly multiple interconnected nodules are present

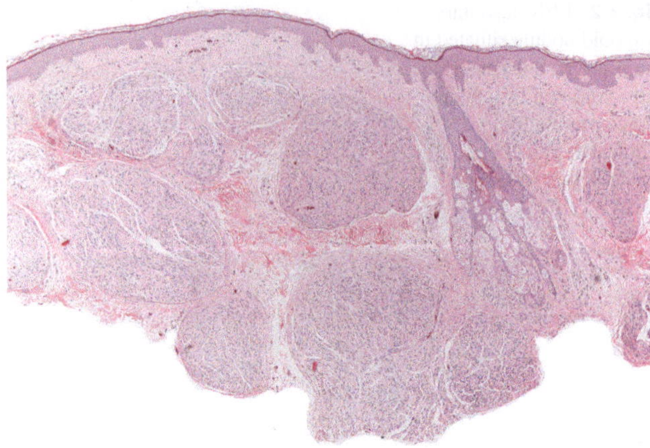

Fig. 3.5 PEN: plexiform variants are rare and composed of numerous interconnected nodules. While not clinically significant, the growth pattern may be confused with schwannoma or neurofibroma

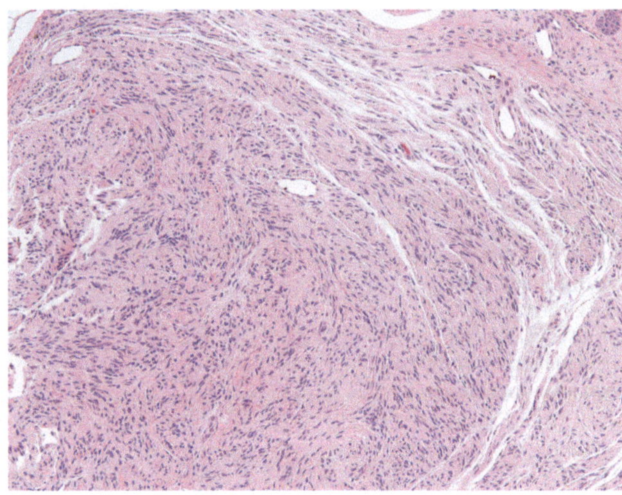

Fig. 3.6 PEN: a typical medium-power appearance showing variably oriented fascicles of Schwann cells separated by clefts

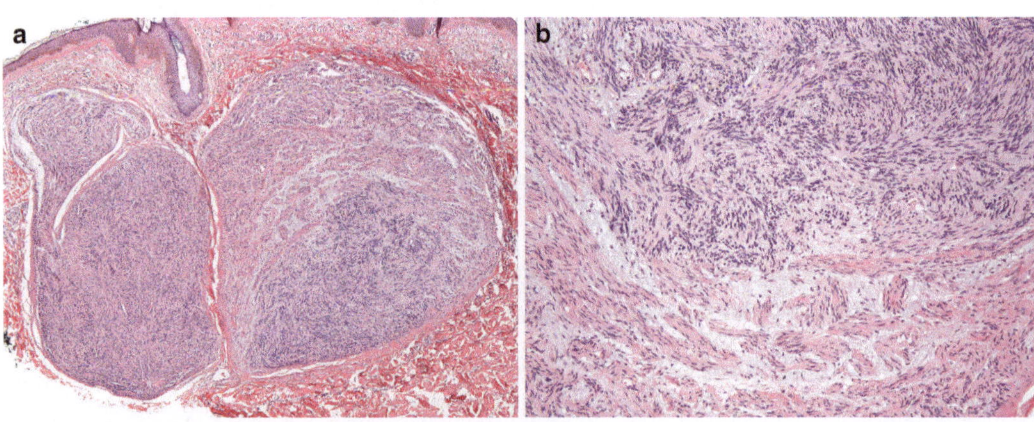

Fig. 3.7 PEN: focal hypercellularity [(**a**) lower right and (**b**) center] may mimic schwannoma. The absence of Verocay bodies and abundance of axons by immunohistochemistry is diagnostic of PEN. Focal myxoid change, an infrequent finding, is also present

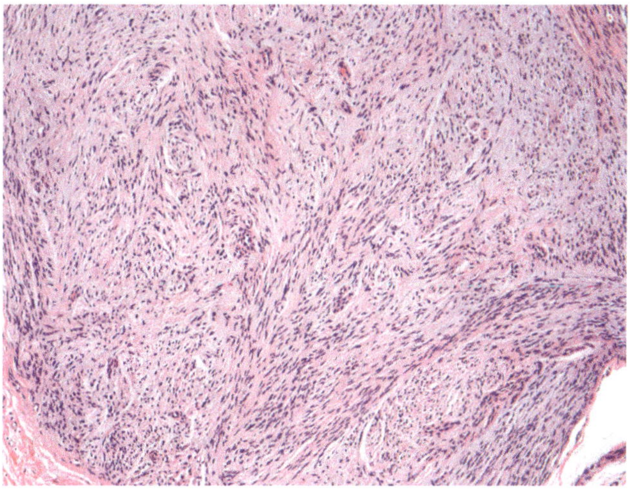

Fig. 3.8 PEN: in some cases, clefts are not prominent between the fascicles. Distinction from schwannoma may require a neurofilaments immunostain

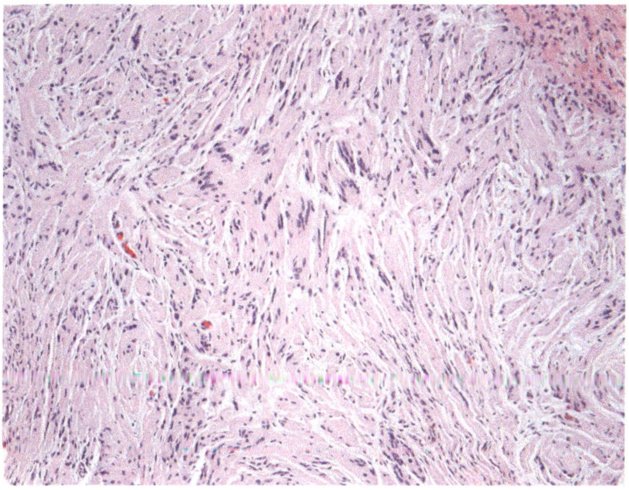

Fig. 3.9 PEN: nuclear palisading may resemble Verocay bodies

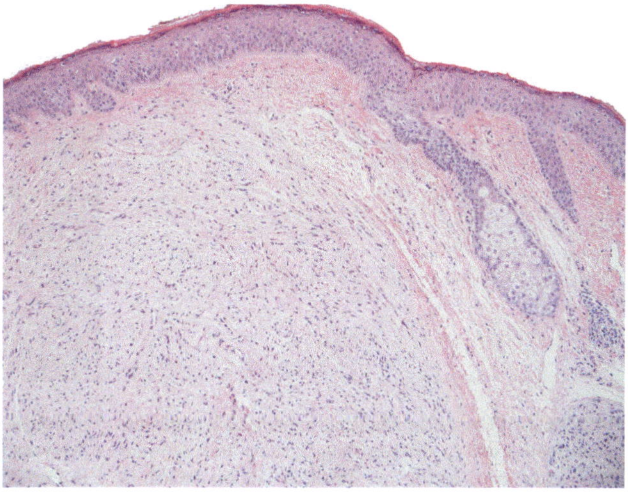

Fig. 3.10 PEN: on occasion, the spindle cells lack fascicular architecture, particularly at the superficial aspect where the mass joins the dermis. This may resemble neurofibroma. Note, however, the thin capsule at the periphery, a characteristic feature of PEN and not neurofibroma

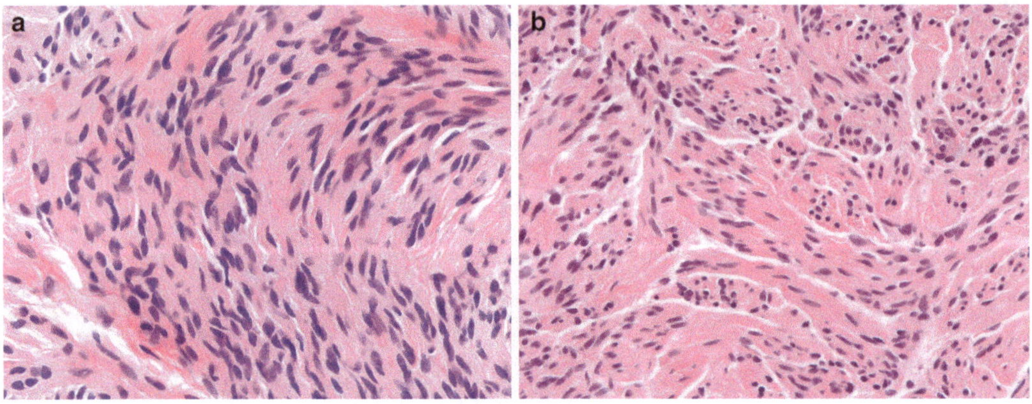

Fig. 3.11 (**a**, **b**) PEN: Schwann cells have uniform slender nuclei with long cytoplasmic processes

Fig. 3.12 PEN: the Schwann cells are uniformly positive for S-100 protein (*red* chromogen)

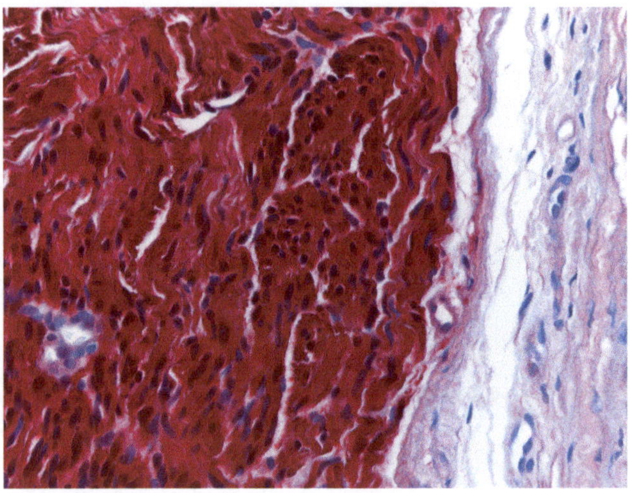

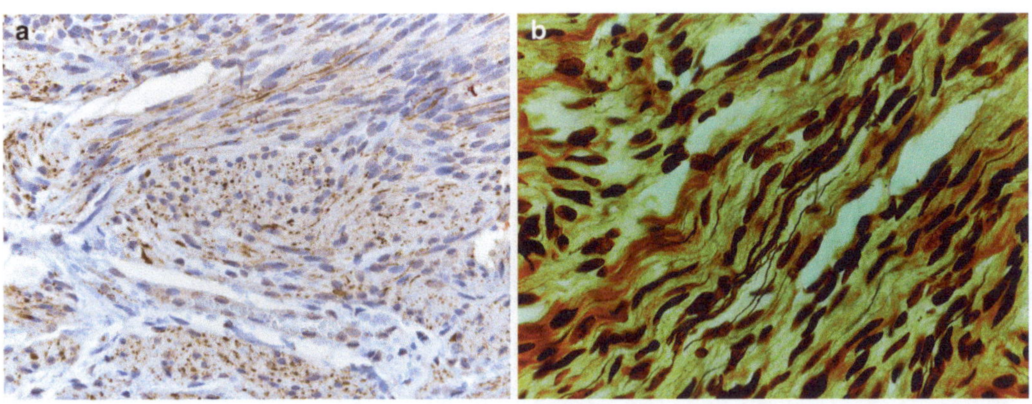

Fig. 3.13 (**a**) PEN: a neurofilaments immunostain highlights innumerable axons, a distinguishing feature from schwannoma where axons are rare or absent. Axons are present in nearly every fascicle and are oriented in the direction of the Schwann cells. When cross-sectioned axons appear as dot-like structures. (**b**) Bielschowsky stain also highlights axons

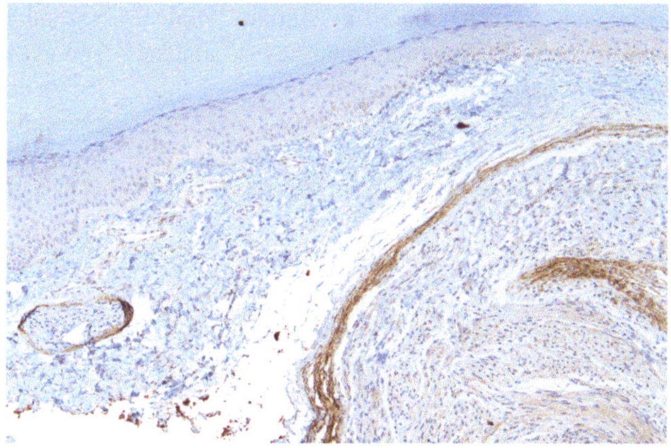

Fig. 3.14 PEN: the perineurial cells surrounding the nodule strongly express epithelial membrane antigen (EMA)

Differential Diagnosis

PEN should be distinguished from other encapsulated dermal neoplasms, such as schwannoma, other neural proliferations including neuromas and neurofibroma, and angioleiomyoma. Like PEN, schwannoma is a circumscribed and encapsulated mass. Both are composed of fascicles of Schwann cells. Most schwannomas however are composed of a mixture of hypercellular and hypocellular areas and without intervening clefts. Verocay bodies are usually present in schwannoma and rare in PEN. A thick collagenous capsule usually surrounds schwannoma in contrast to the thin layer of perineurium around PEN. The presence of numerous axons can be an important distinguishing factor as axons are rare or absent in schwannoma. Not all fascicles within PEN contain abundant axons, so one must carefully examine the entire lesion. Plexiform PEN specifically mimics plexiform schwannoma, as both are hypercellular; in these cases, a neurofilaments immunostain is often contributory. Mucosal neuroma can closely mimic PEN and correlation with clinical findings is necessary. In most cases, however, mucosal neuroma does not form a well-defined large nodular mass-like PEN, but rather comprises multiple variably expanded nerve fascicles and fibers. The organized pattern of intersecting fascicles separated by prominent clefts is lacking in mucosal neuroma. In large mucosal neuromas, individual nerve fascicles are recognizable, opposed to the hypercellular fascicles of PEN. Neurofibroma in most cases is readily separated from PEN by its (usually) disordered and haphazardly arrangement of Schwann cells, the presence of other cells including dendritic cells, polygonal cells, and inflammatory cells. Neurofibroma contains much fewer sparse axons that lack the parallel arrangements to the direction of the fascicle seen in PEN. Tumors with circumscribed nodular proliferations of nonneural origin should also be excluded. This includes angioleiomyoma, which is composed of abundant vessels and smooth muscle cells and lacks a Schwann cell population, as confirmed by reactivity with immunostains like smooth muscle actin, desmin, and CD31.

Mucosal (Mucocutaneous) Neuroma

Definition, Classification, and Histogenesis

Mucosal or mucocutaneous neuromas are hamartomas that often occur in patients with MEN type 2B and rarely in PTEN mutation-associated hamartoma syndromes. Like PEN, mucosal neuroma arises without antecedent trauma.

Clinical

Mucosal neuromas show a strong predilection for the perioral skin and oral mucosa. Lesions may be solitary or multiple that latter in patients with MEN. They appear as flesh-colored papules.

Individual lesions share a similar clinical appearance to PEN, intradermal nevus, adnexal tumors, or basal cell carcinoma.

Histopathology

Mucosal neuromas are composed of multiple variably enlarged individual nerve fibers and fascicles in the superficial dermis or subepithelial stroma (Figs. 3.15–3.19). The fascicles resemble normal nerve, are composed of Schwann cells and axons, and surrounded by perineurium. The lesion may form a well-defined mass, but in many cases, multiple individual fascicles are present in a somewhat disordered manner. Dermal fibrosis may be present but marked scarring and inflammation is absent (Figs. 3.20–3.22). Similar proliferations may be encountered in skin not adjacent to a mucosal site and likely represent a similar hamartomatous process (Figs. 3.23 and 3.24).

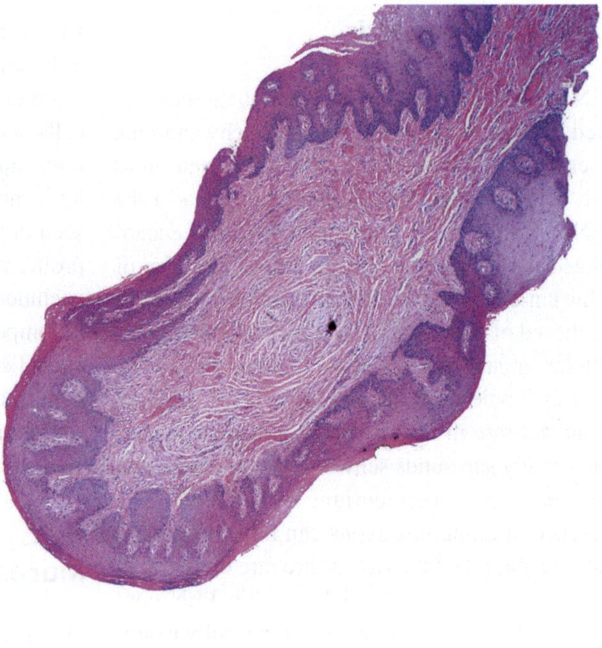

Fig. 3.15 Mucosal (mucocutaneous) neuroma: a polypoid piece of squamous mucosa from the mouth with hyperkeratosis, epithelial hyperplasia, and a somewhat circumscribed, unencapsulated proliferation of nerve fascicles in the stroma

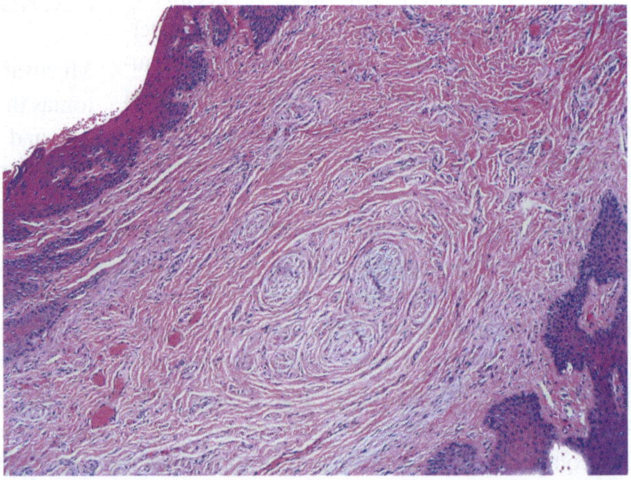

Fig. 3.16 Mucosal neuroma: individual fascicles of varying size are surrounded by dense collagen. The proliferation lacks the dense fibrosis and inflammation of traumatic neuroma

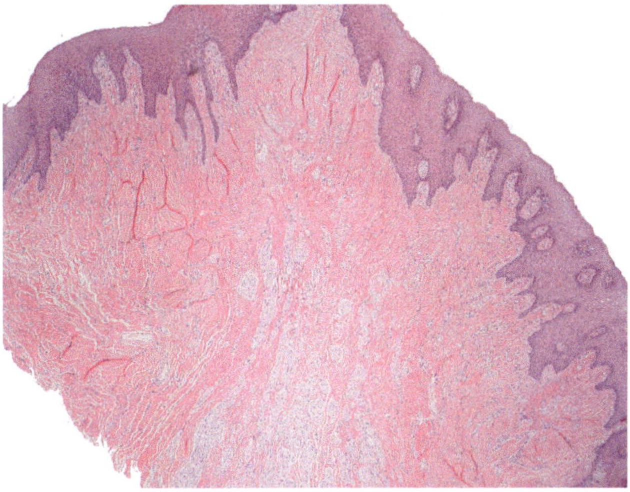

Fig. 3.17 Mucosal neuroma: this oral lesion shows a more prominent defined proliferation of nerve fascicles in the stroma

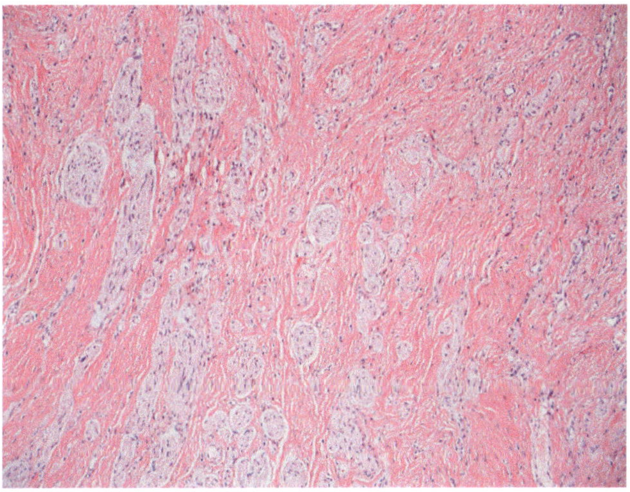

Fig. 3.18 Mucosal neuroma: individual fascicles of varying size are surrounded by dense collagen (higher magnification)

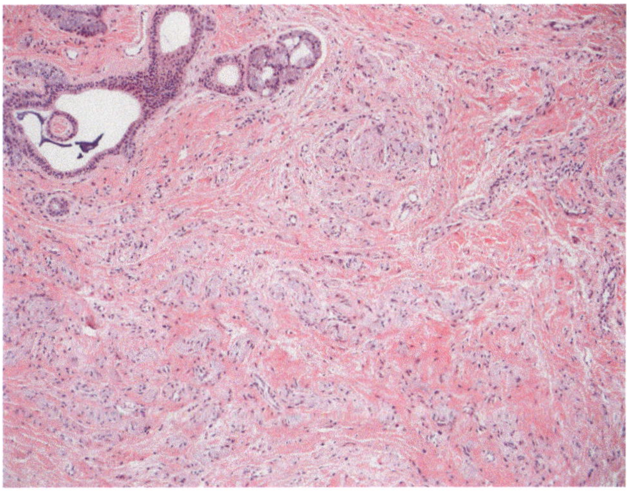

Fig. 3.19 Mucosal neuroma: small nerve fascicles are adjacent to minor salivary glands. The proliferation lacks the dense fibrosis and inflammation of traumatic neuroma

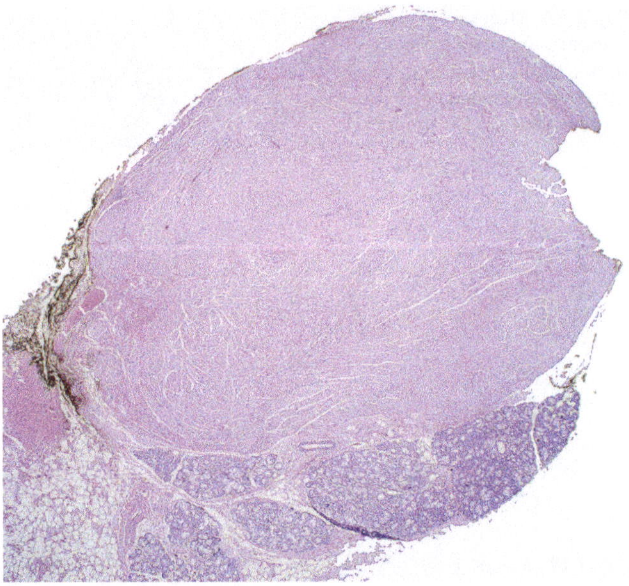

Fig. 3.20 Mucosal neuroma: some lesions present as a large circumscribed mass. This example from the lip is adjacent to minor salivary gland. The mass is unencapsulated, a distinguishing feature from PEN

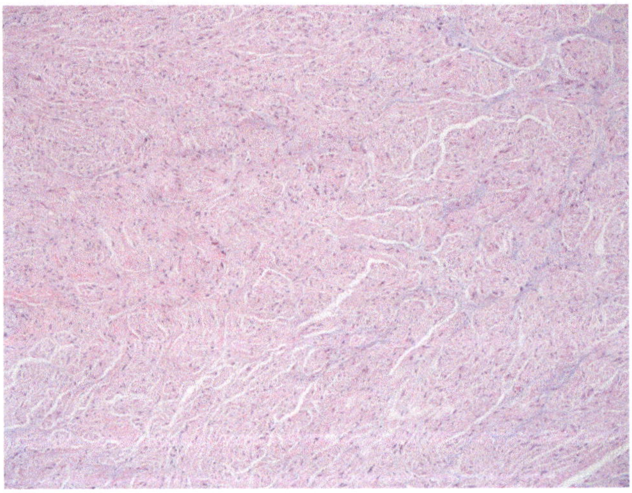

Fig. 3.21 Mucocutaneous neuroma: fascicles of variable size are closely opposed, separated by basophilic mucinous material. The clefts mimic those of PEN

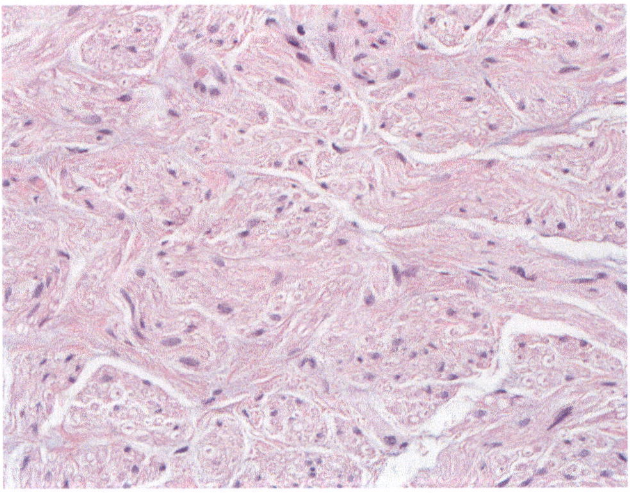

Fig. 3.22 Mucocutaneous neuroma: at higher magnification, the fascicles closely resemble normal nerve with prominent axons, in contrast to the Schwann cell rich nature of PEN

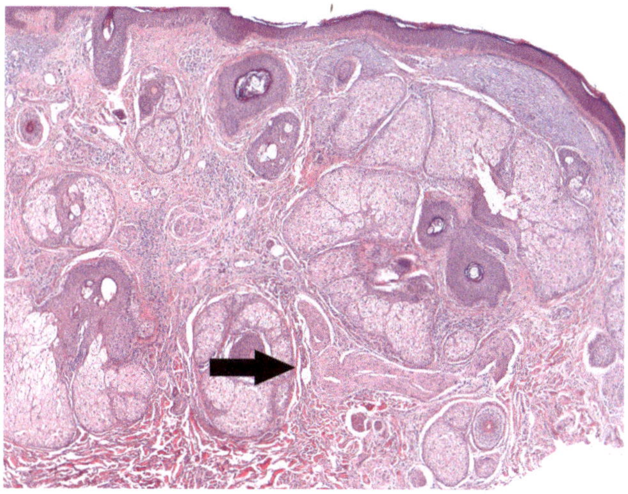

Fig. 3.23 Linear neuroma, also known as *solitary neural hamartoma*: a large tortuous nerve fascicle adjacent to prominent sebaceous glands (*arrow*)

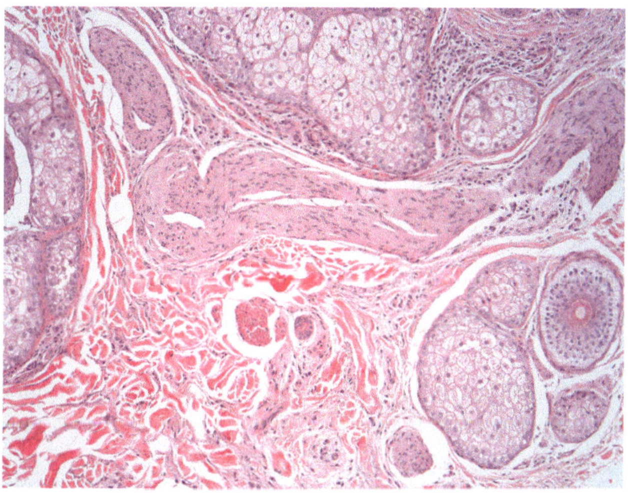

Fig. 3.24 Linear neuroma, also known as *solitary neural hamartoma*: a large tortuous nerve fascicle adjacent to prominent sebaceous glands (higher magnification)

Differential Diagnosis

The main distinction is from PEN and traumatic neuroma. Clinically, the presence of multiple perioral lesions is most suggestive of mucosal neuroma. Histopathologically, mucosal neuroma usually does not form a distinct nodule like PEN; however, if present, mucosal neuroma lacks a true capsule and is composed of individual structures resembling nerve fascicles, rather than nodules of spindle cells arranged in intersecting fascicles separated by clefts. Traumatic neuroma is usually distinguished by clinical history. Like mucocutaneous neuroma is a seemingly haphazard proliferation of variably sized nerve fibers and fascicles; however, traumatic neuroma usually has a more disordered appearance with a heavily fibrotic or inflamed stroma.

Fibrolipomatous Hamartoma

Definition, Classification, and Histogenesis

Fibrolipomatous hamartoma (FLH) is not in actuality a neural proliferation. Rather, it is an overgrowth of fibroadipose tissue within a large peripheral nerve. FLH may represent a hamartoma of the epineurium. Synonyms include *lipomatosis of nerve*, *intraneural lipoma*, and *neural fibrolipoma*.

Clinical

FLH most commonly affects young adults. The median nerve is most commonly involved. As such, FLH usually presents as unilateral expansion of the volar forearm at the wrist, palm, finger, or a combination of the above. The digits may appear clinically enlarged. Most involve the deep soft tissues although on occasion large lesions may protrude into the superficial tissues. Median nerve lesions may be a source of carpal tunnel syndrome in children.

Histopathology

FLH is composed of abundant mature fibroadipose tissue within the epineurium. The lobules of fat surround and separate the residual nerve fascicles. There may be increased collagen deposition of the perineurium or endoneurium, but inflammation is uncommon (Figs. 3.25 and 3.26).

Differential Diagnosis

None if completely resected. Partial biopsy may be misdiagnosed as lipoma.

Traumatic Neuroma

Definition, Classification, and Histogenesis

Traumatic neuromas are regenerative hyperplastic proliferations of nerve in response to injury. Following transection of a nerve, there is Wallerian degeneration of the proximal aspect with an attempt by the distal portion to reconnect to the opposite end. This results in a disorganized proliferation of nerve fibers, usually in the dermis. Amputation neuromas are etiologically similar attempts at nerve regeneration following transection (see Fig. 3.27a, b for line drawing). Supernumerary digits (rudimentary polydactyly) are not true neuromas but an embryologic remnant of multiple cutaneous elements including nerve, presumably due to incomplete apoptosis in utero.

Clinical

Traumatic neuroma presents as a dermal nodule or mass, often on the acral skin and digits. Lesions are often painful and associated with abnormal sensations such as phantom pain. Penile lesions may resemble condyloma.

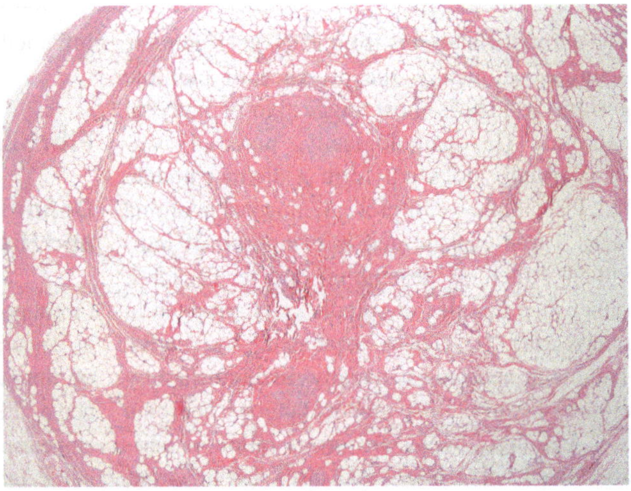

Fig. 3.25 Fibrolipomatous hamartoma: the median nerve is surrounded by abundant lobules of mature adipose tissue separated by collagen. The fibroadipose tissue presumably arises from epineurium

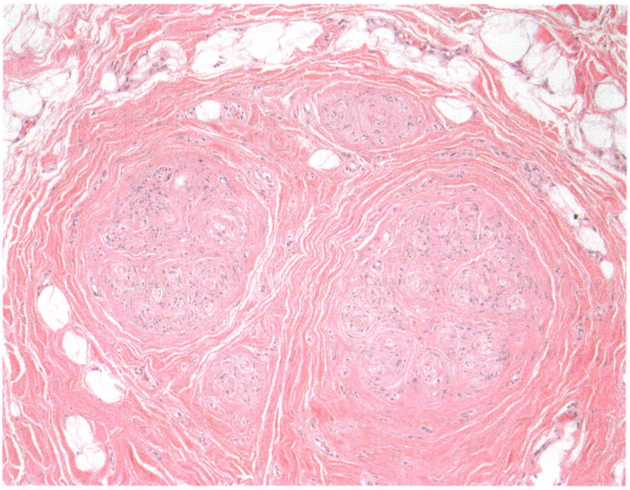

Fig. 3.26 Fibrolipomatous hamartoma: although there is expansion of the epineurium, the nerve fascicles and fibers are unremarkable

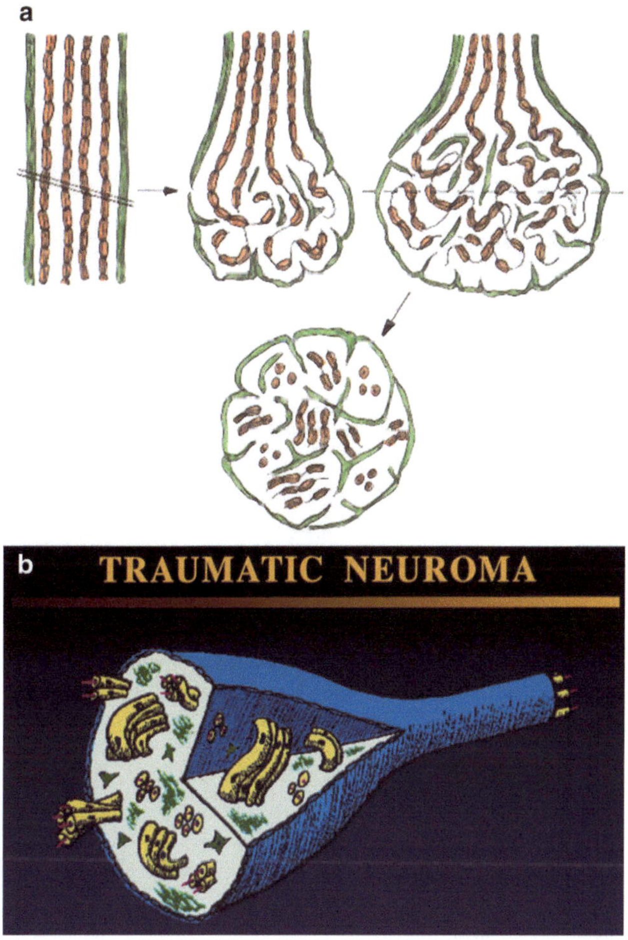

Fig. 3.27 (**a**, **b**) Schematic drawing of *traumatic neuroma*: individual fascicles proliferate in a haphazard manner in response to traumatic injury. There is disruption of the perineurium (artwork by ZA)

Histopathology

Traumatic neuroma is an unorganized mass of small and large nerve fibers composed of each of the nerve elements – Schwann cells, axons, and perineurial cells (Figs. 3.28–3.30). The surrounding dermis shows reparative changes including inflammation, granulation tissue, fibrosis, and scar corresponding with the duration of the lesion (Fig. 3.31). The epidermis may be acanthotic. Amputation neuromas are large deep masses with similar findings. The larger branches of nerve may be mucin rich especially around the perineurium. In traumatic neuromas of small peripheral nerves, the small, disorganized fibers are in continuity with the surrounding dermis. In contrast, a dense fibrous pseudocapsule is often present around amputation neuromas involving larger nerve branches (Figs. 3.32–3.34). The histologic findings in supernumerary digits are similar (Figs. 3.35 and 3.36).

Differential Diagnosis

Clinical history is contributory, notable for trauma or recent surgery. The presence of multiple disorganized nerve fibers in a dense fibrous and

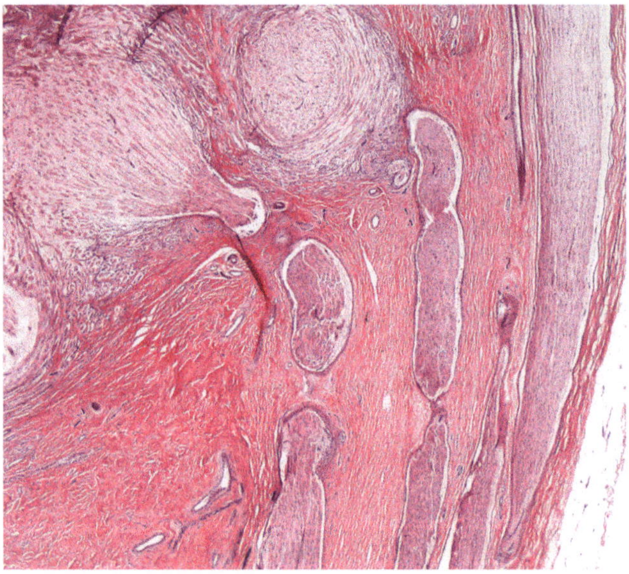

Fig. 3.28 Traumatic neuroma: a large injured nerve (*right*) and a reactive proliferation of smaller fascicles (*left*) with marked fibrosis and myxoid change is characteristic

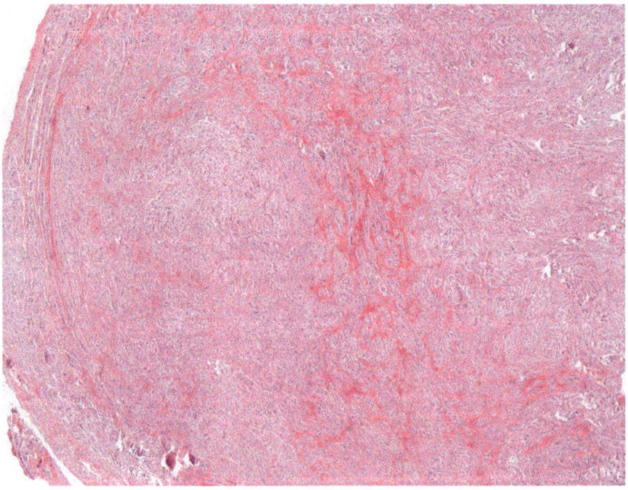

Fig. 3.29 Traumatic neuroma: the proliferation may result in a well-circumscribed mass resembling a neoplasm

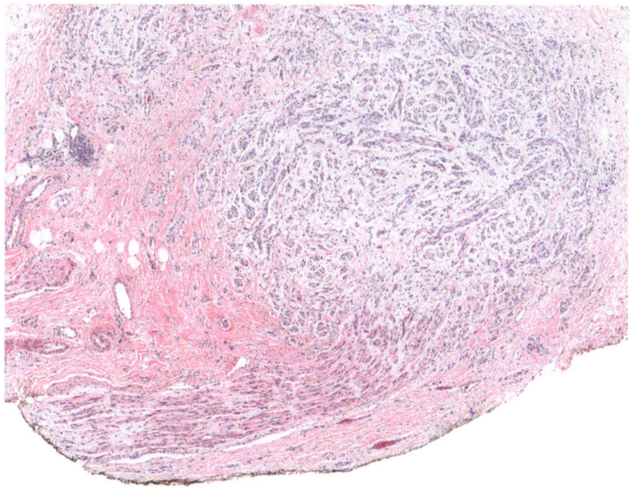

Fig. 3.30 Traumatic neuroma: small fibers and fascicles proliferate from the larger parent fascicles

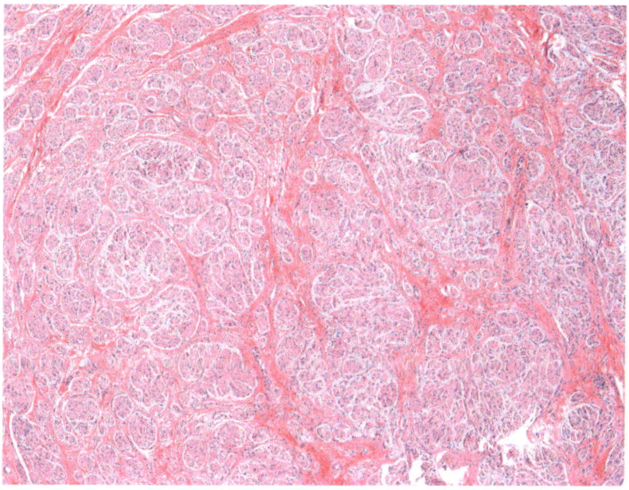

Fig. 3.31 Traumatic neuroma: the nerve fascicles may form lobules separated by fibrous tissue

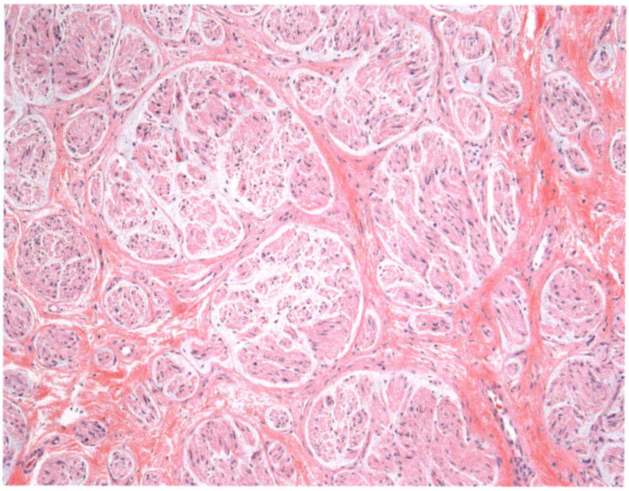

Fig. 3.32 Traumatic neuroma: fascicles are composed of Schwann cells and axons, resembling those of mucosal neuroma

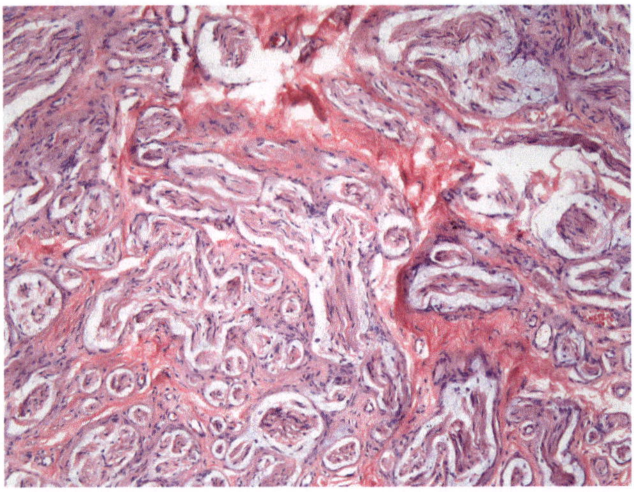

Fig. 3.33 Traumatic neuroma: mucin often separates the individual fascicles

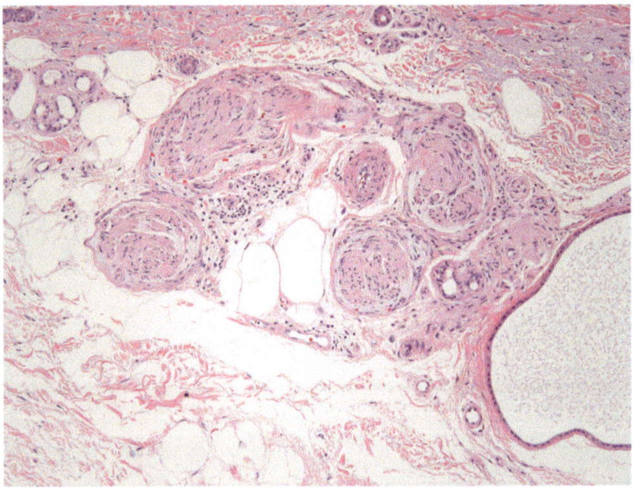

Fig. 3.34 Traumatic neuroma: a small abnormal nerve in an excisional biopsy of a basal cell carcinoma represents early changes of traumatic neuroma. There is early disorganization of nerve fibers within the fascicles and focal mucin deposition

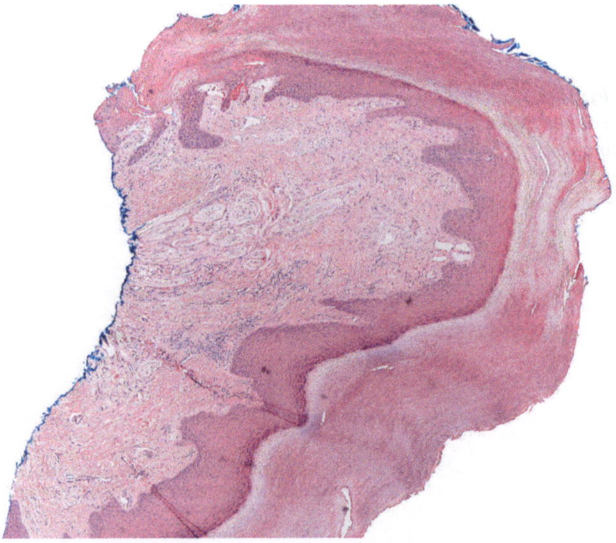

Fig. 3.35 Supernumerary digit: a polypoid portion of acral skin with small nodular aggregate of nerve fascicles in the dermis. These are likely the result of incomplete apoptosis in utero

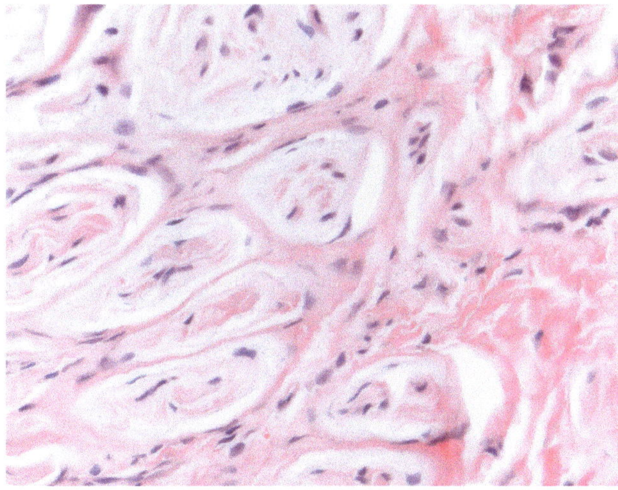

Fig. 3.36 Supernumerary digit: nerve fascicles are small and are disorganized within the lobular configuration

inflamed stroma separates traumatic neuroma from PEN and mucosal neuroma and can easily be confirmed by traditional silver stain (Bodian or Bielschowsky) or neural filament immunostain.

Morton's Neuroma (Interdigital Neuritis)

Definition, Classification, and Histogenesis

Morton's neuroma is a common inflammatory and fibrosing disorder of peripheral nerve. It is a reactive response to chronic injury or irritation and not a neoplasm or hamartoma; however, it is discussed here for historic purposes.

Clinical

Morton's neuroma usually arises on the plantar surfaces of the foot, affecting the nerves between the second and third or third and fourth toes. It is nearly always unilateral and common in women who wear high-heel shoes. Patients report pain when walking that improves with rest.

Histopathology

The excisional specimen has a characteristic fusiform appearance at low power and is identifiable as a peripheral nerve. Within the nerve, there is fibrosis of the perineurium. The residual nerve fascicles often have a nodular appearance within the substance of the nerve secondary to the abundant collagen. The fibrosis may involve the epineurium and extend into the adjacent fibroadipose tissue. Mucin deposition may be present. Vessels are often increased and have thickened walls. A mild lymphocytic infiltrate may be present (Figs. 3.37–3.39).

Differential Diagnosis

Morton's neuroma may resemble traumatic neuroma but differs on both clinical and histopathologic grounds. Unlike traumatic neuroma, Morton's neuroma lacks the multiple small fascicles common to the former. Also, the fibrosis in Morton's neuroma is present within and around the nerve, while in traumatic neuroma, the adjacent dermis is fibrotic. Inflammation may be present in both.

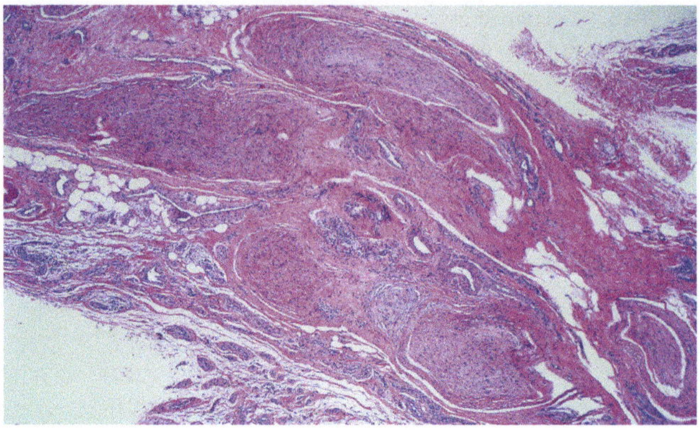

Fig. 3.37 Morton's neuroma: a fusiform mass representing residual nerve in which there is marked fibrosis and patchy inflammation

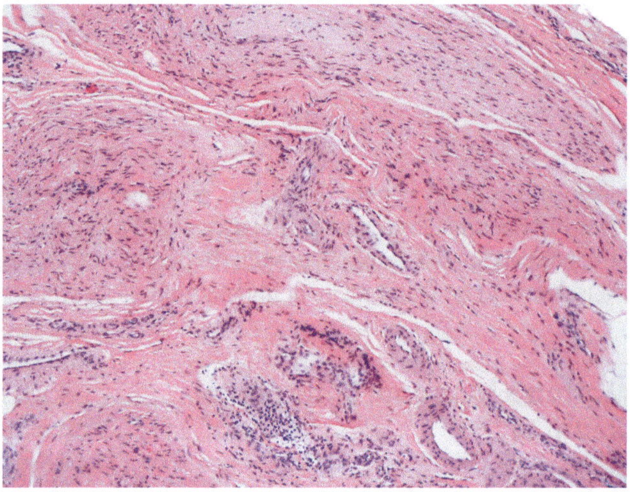

Fig. 3.38 Morton's neuroma: the fascicles are recognized as such but are distorted by the prominent fibrosis

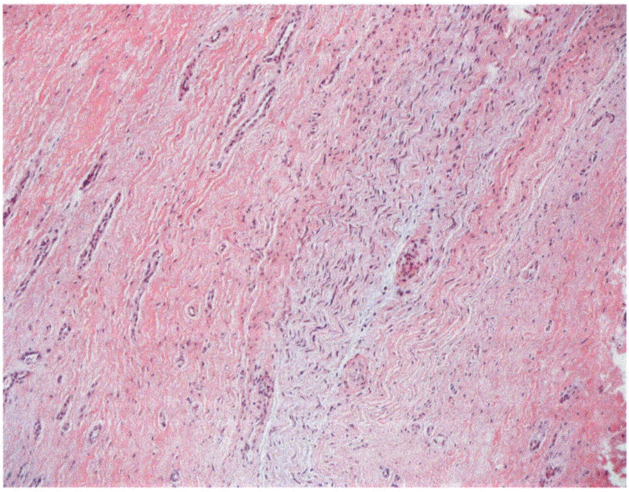

Fig. 3.39 Morton's neuroma: small vessels are often increased in the fibrous tissue and may have a hyalinized appearance

Reparative Perineurial Hyperplasia

Definition, Classification, and Histogenesis

Reparative perineurial cell hyperplasia is a reactive proliferation of perineurial cells around residual nerves within an area of skin subjected to surgery or biopsy. The histopathologic features can closely mimic perineurial spread of an epithelial neoplasm like squamous cell carcinoma.

Clinical

Perineurial hyperplasia is an incidental histopathologic finding and not a clinically evident lesion.

Histopathology

Following injury or surgical manipulation, perineurial cells enlarge and proliferate around otherwise normal appearing nerves in the dermis. The perineurial cells are plump and polygonal or spindled and form concentric one to three cells thick layers. The perineurial cells are positive for EMA and negative for cytokeratins. Reparative changes in the adjacent dermis including inflammation, granulation tissue, or fibrosis are usually evident (Figs. 3.40–3.42).

Differential Diagnosis

The increased nuclear size and location around the periphery of the nerve resembles squamous cell carcinoma with perineurial spread. The presence of these cells within or adjacent to scar or granulation tissue, and expression of EMA without expression of cytokeratins distinguish it from carcinoma.

Epithelial Sheath Neuroma

Definition, Classification, and Histogenesis

Epithelial sheath neuroma is a histopathologic entity characterized by enlarged dermal nerve fibers surrounded by epithelium. The exact etiology of this lesion is debated. The authors who first described this lesion believed it was a neoplasm, but others contend it represents an unusual hyperplastic phenomenon secondary to injury like chronic mechanical irritation or a ruptured cyst. The peripheral layer of epithelium may be derived from the adjacent epidermis or infundibulum.

Clinical

Epithelial sheath neuroma presents as small papules on the back of older adults. The papules may be painful, pruritic, or asymptomatic.

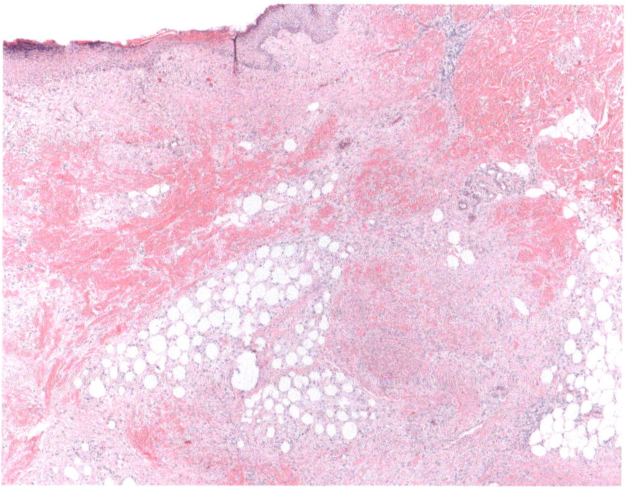

Fig. 3.40 Reparative perineurial cell hyperplasia: a biopsy site with superficial granulation tissue and fibrosis, patchy lymphocytic inflammation, and fat necrosis. The entrapped nerve fascicles in the deep dermis and subcutis have an expanded layer of perineurial cells

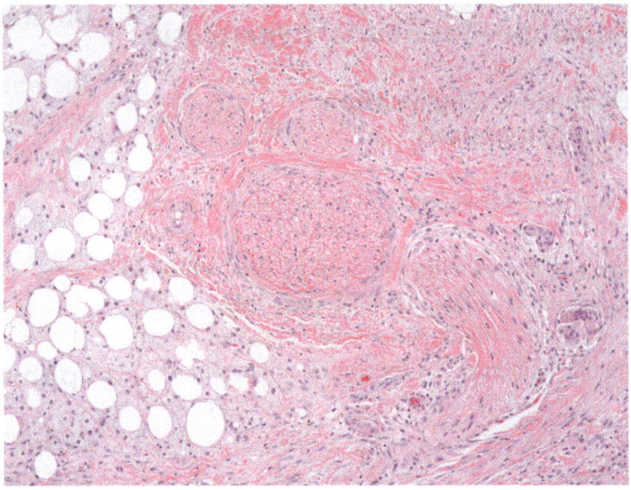

Fig. 3.41 Reparative perineurial cell hyperplasia: concentric layers of perineurial cells surround each fascicle. These may mimic perineurial spread of squamous cell carcinoma

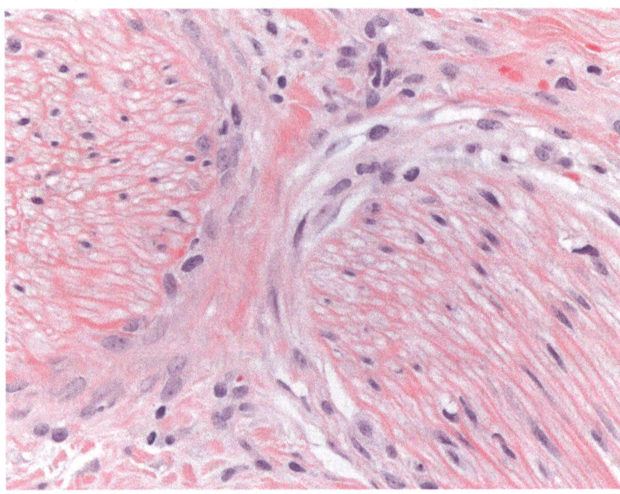

Fig. 3.42 Reparative perineurial cell hyperplasia: the perineurial cells are spindled to slightly polygonal, mimicking squamous cell carcinoma. There is no significant pleomorphism, however, and the perineurial cells appear to merge with each other, lacking well-defined borders. Carcinoma is also not identified in the adjacent dermis. Expression of EMA and absence of cytokeratins may also aid in excluding malignancy

Histopathology

Epithelial sheath neuroma consists of expanded nerve fibers in the superficial dermis, each of which is encompassed by a sheath of squamous epithelium. The expanded nerves are large compared to normal fascicles in the superficial dermis and are arranged in a haphazard manner. Otherwise they are composed of the typical elements. There may be an adjacent lymphocyte infiltrate. Small infundibular cysts may be present nearby, suggesting the epithelial sheaths derive from the follicular infundibulum. Occasional dyskeratotic cells may be present. There is no associated fibrosis but myxoid change may be observed (Figs. 3.43 and 3.44)

Differential Diagnosis

The histologic findings are unique and identifiable as such. Lesions may mimic perineurial involvement by an epithelial malignancy. The lack of keratinocyte nuclear atypia and orderly maturation argues against a squamous neoplasm. While the disordered appearance of fascicles may resemble traumatic neuroma, the latter lacks an epithelial sheath and is associated with dermal fibrosis.

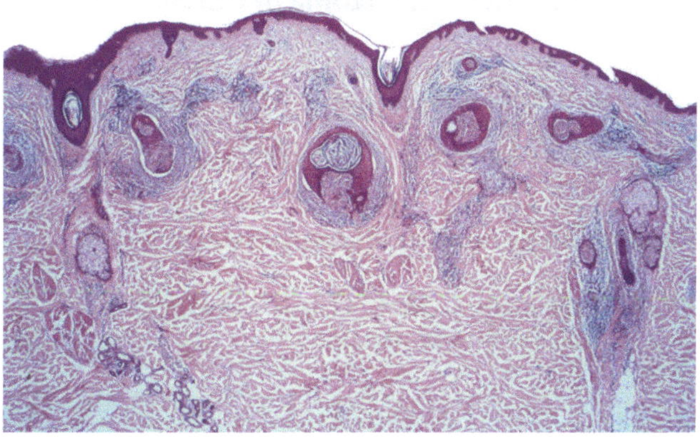

Fig. 3.43 Epithelial sheath neuroma: multiple rather large nerve fibers in the superficial dermis are surrounded by epithelium. Many are present near folliculosebaceous units. There is an adjacent lymphocytic infiltrate. Courtesy of Drs. L. Requena and H. Kutzner

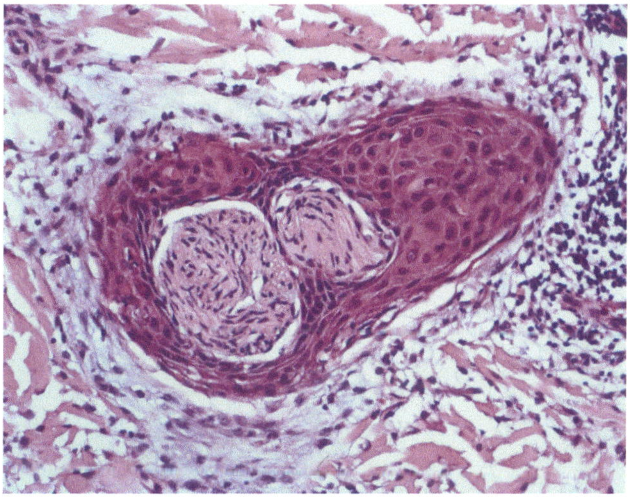

Fig. 3.44 Epithelial sheath neuroma: the nerve fibers are enlarged for their location in the dermis but otherwise morphologically unremarkable. The surrounding sheath of squamous cells is cytologically bland. Courtesy of Drs. L. Requena and H. Kutzner

Additional Reading

Palisaded Encapsulated Neuroma

Argenyi ZB. Immunohistochemical characterization of palisaded, encapsulated neuroma. J Cutan Pathol. 1990;17:329.

Argenyi ZB, Santa Cruz D, Bromley C. Comparative light-microscopic and immunohistochemical study of traumatic and palisaded encapsulated neuromas of the skin. Am J Dermatopathol. 1992;14:504.

Argenyi ZB, Cooper PH, Santa Cruz D. Plexiform and other unusual variants of palisaded encapsulated neuroma. J Cutan Pathol. 1993;20:34.

Fletcher CDM. Solitary circumscribed neuroma of the skin (so-called palisaded, encapsulated neuroma). A clinicopathologic and immunohistochemical study. Am J Surg Pathol. 1989;13:574.

Jokinen CH, Ragsdale BD, Argenyi ZB. Expanding the clinicopathologic spectrum of palisaded encapsulated neuroma. J Cutan Pathol. 2010;37:43.

Reed RJ, Fine RM, Meltzer HD. Palisaded, encapsulated neuromas of the skin. Arch Dermatol. 1972; 106:865.

Mucosal Neuroma

Gorlin RJ, Sedano HO, Vickers RA, Cervenka J. Multiple mucosal neuromas, pheochromocytoma and medullary carcinoma of the thyroid – a syndrome. Cancer. 1968;22:293.

Schaffer JV, Kamino H, Witkiewicz A, McNiff JM, Orlow SJ. Mucocutaneous neuromas: an underrecognized manifestation of PTEN hamartoma-tumor syndrome. Arch Dermatol. 2006;142:625.

Fibrolipomatous Hamartoma of Nerve

Silverman TA, Enzinger FM. Fibrolipomatous hamartoma of nerve. A clinicopathologic analysis of 26 cases. Am J Surg Pathol. 1985;9:7.

Reparative Perineurial Hyperplasia

Beer TW. Reparative perineural hyperplasia: a series of 10 cases. Am J Dermatopathol. 2009;31:50.

Epithelial Sheath Neuroma

Requena L, Grosshans E, Kutzner H, et al. Epithelial sheath neuroma: a new entity. Am J Surg Pathol. 2000;24:190.

Zelger BG, Zelger B. Epithelial sheath neuroma: a benign neoplasm? Am J Surg Pathol. 2001;25:696.

Benign Cutaneous Neoplasms with Peripheral Nerve Differentiation

4

Keywords
Benign cutaneous neural neoplasms • Classification • Histogenesis • Diagnostic features • Differential diagnosis • Common neurofibroma • Neurofibroma variants • Common schwannoma • Schwannoma variants • Granular cell tumor • Nerve sheath myxoma • Perineurioma • Lipoblastic nerve sheath tumors

Neurofibroma

Definition, Classification, and Histogenesis

Neurofibroma (NF) is one of the most commonly encountered benign peripheral nerve sheath tumors in the skin (Fig. 4.1a, b for line drawing). Because NF is composed of each element of the peripheral nerve, it most likely represents a hamartoma. Some authors, however, contend NF is a neoplasm as it is associated with mutation in the neurofibromatosis type 1 (NF1) gene. Furthermore, neurofibroma may undergo malignant transformation to malignant peripheral nerve sheath tumor. This occurs most often in patients with NF1.

Clinical Findings

Cutaneous neurofibroma may occur at any site. Solitary lesions are most common and present as skin-colored, soft, rubbery, or firm papules or nodules. Clinically, most show no epidermal changes unless there is trauma, which often occurs on the extremities. These resemble intradermal nevi or when pedunculated, soft fibromas (skin tags). Multiple cutaneous lesions may be seen in NF1. Plexiform NF is less common in the skin and usually found in the deeper soft tissues, where it is strongly indicative of NF1. When it manifests as such, it is characterized by large cord, nodular, or bag-like soft tissue masses with predilection on the buttocks and trunk. They are usually skin-colored, but hyperpigmented macules and patches can be associated. For detailed discussion of neurofibromatosis as a genetically determined clinicopathologic entity, the reader is referred to relevant literature.

Histopathology

Neurofibromas are nonencapsulated proliferations of multiple cell types in a variably collagenous and myxoid stroma. Numerous histopathologic variants of neurofibroma are described, the most common of which are solitary (Fig. 4.2) and diffuse (Fig. 4.3). These variants are summarized in Table 4.1. In general, each shares the same immunohistochemical profile.

Solitary NF is commonly a sporadic proliferation that is well delineated from the surrounding dermis, but lacks a capsule (Figs. 4.4 and 4.5).

Z. Argenyi and C.H. Jokinen (eds.), *Cutaneous Neural Neoplasms*, Current Clinical Pathology,
DOI 10.1007/978-1-60327-582-8_4, © Springer Science+Business Media, LLC 2011

a

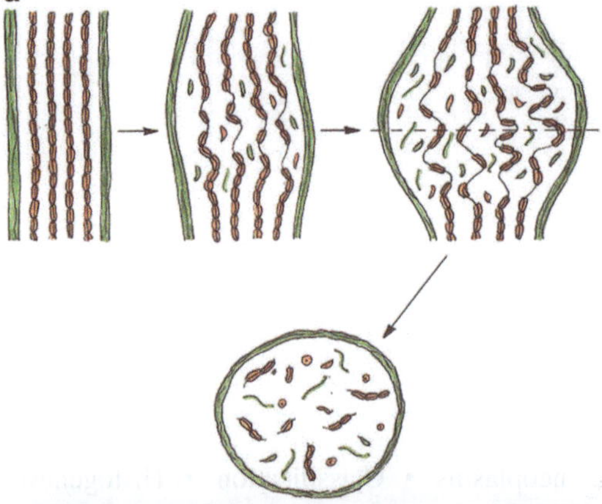

b

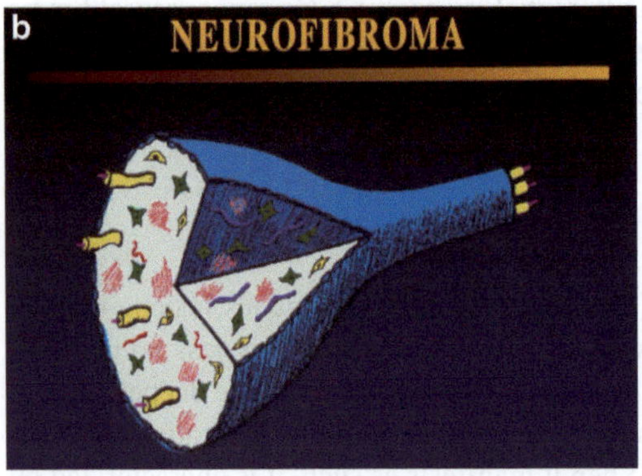

Fig. 4.1 (**a**, **b**) Schematic representations of *neurofibroma*. There is heterogeneous expansion of the nerve by multiple cell populations, collagen, and mucopolysaccharide-rich stroma. Elements of the nerve fascicle including Schwann cells, axons, and intraneural stromal cells like fibrocytes in addition to inflammatory cells are present. Conceptually, NF develops from within the nerve fascicle as a hamartoma, whereas schwannoma (Fig. 4.38) develops eccentrically from the nerve from a single neoplastic cell (artwork by ZA)

On a low magnification, it often shows a nodular or polypoid growth pattern. The predominant cell is the Schwann cell, which has a small thin spindled nucleus with wavy contours and fine chromatin. Nucleoli are often inconspicuous. The Schwann cells have fine fibrillar cytoplasmic processes (Figs. 4.6 and 4.7). These are haphazardly arranged and admixed with small polygonal cells, mast cells, and dendritic cells. Often the Schwann cells are arranged in short bundles with dense collagen known as the shredded carrot pattern. The Schwann cells strongly express nuclear and cytoplasmic S-100 protein (Fig. 4.8). It should be noted that unlike schwannoma, only a portion of the cells in neurofibromas are S-100 protein positive, however, which gives a somewhat "spotty or loose" staining pattern, quite different from the diffuse reactivity seen in schwannoma or neuroma. Silver impregnation also highlights scattered axons (Figs. 4.9 and 4.10). A subset of cells will stain with CD34. Epithelial membrane antigen (EMA) will stain perineurial cells if present in the surrounding tissue, and may stain few cells in the peripheral portions of the mass. A neurofilament stain will highlight axons haphazardly present in the stroma. In some cases, this immunostain may identify residual or entrapped nerve fibers. Schwann cells are either haphazardly arranged, or may form vague hypocellular fascicles. *Diffuse NF* lacks the well-circumscribed nature of solitary forms. The cellular composition is identical in each however.

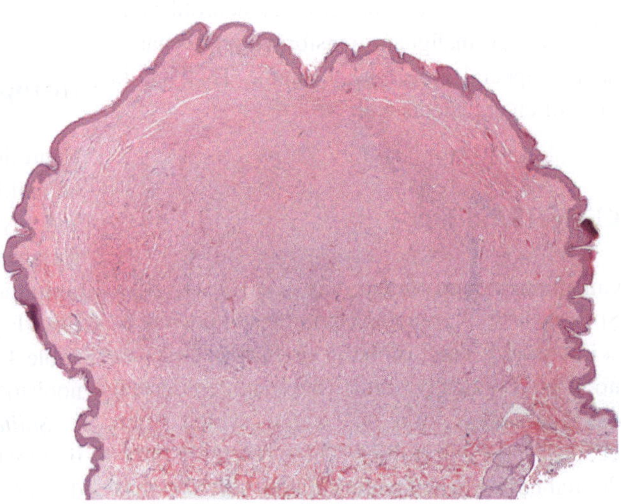

Fig. 4.2 Solitary neurofibroma: a commonly encountered form is a polypoid soft nodule due to a superficial dermal proliferation. The mass is nonencapsulated but well circumscribed with uninvolved dermis between the mass and epidermis

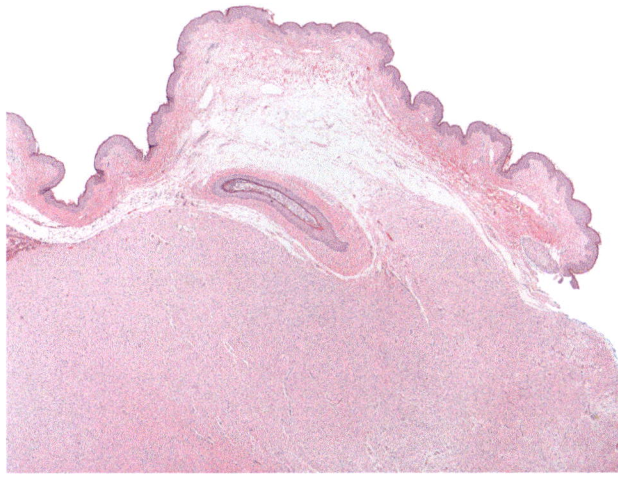

Fig. 4.3 Neurofibroma with a *diffuse* growth pattern: a proliferation extends from the subcutis into the superficial aspects of the skin

Table 4.1 Neurofibroma variants

Solitary
Diffuse
Plexiform
Dendritic cell neurofibroma with pseudorosettes
Atypical/cellular
Pigmented
Myxoid
Epithelioid
Perineurioma-like

Often small blood vessels are admixed with the neural components. Diffuse NF may infiltrate the surrounding tissue such as adipose tissue or skeletal muscle. *Plexiform NF* is composed of multiple nodules and cord-like structures, likely representing tortuous growth of involved individual nerve fascicles sectioned in multiple planes (see line drawing, Fig. 4.11). The nodules can present in a background of a diffuse neurofibroma. In larger and clinically more evident nodular and bag-like lesions, the plexiform pattern can be even visible on gross examination as interconnected string or mop-like structures (Fig. 4.12). The internal growth pattern and cytologic features of solitary, diffuse, and plexiform forms of neurofibromas are similar (Figs. 4.13 and 4.14). Growth around nerves is often evident (Fig. 4.15). In diffuse forms, Schwann cell rich nodules may occur, resembling structures otherwise seen in schwannoma (Fig. 4.16). NF may manifest structures resembling Meissner corpuscles (pseudomeissnerian bodies) (Fig. 4.17a, b). These closely resemble the so-called neurotization that commonly occurs in melanocytic nevi (Fig. 4.18a, b).

Dendritic cell neurofibroma is a rare, recently described variant of neurofibroma with lobular growth pattern containing rosette-like structures with centrally located dendrite-like large vacuolated cells (Figs. 4.19–4.21).

Atypical or *cellular NF* is a rare morphologic variant that may present a diagnostic challenge (Figs. 4.22 and 4.23). Often, but not always, increased cellularity and nuclear atypia or pleomorphism are seen together and will be discussed as such here. Atypical cells in these variants often comprise the minority of cells and are intermixed with the more typical cells of NF (Fig. 4.24). The atypical cells are often quite large, hyperchromatic, have irregular nuclear contours, and may have a vacuolated nuclear appearance or well-defined pseudoinclusions. Sometimes there is a sharply delineated cytoplasm unlike the typical Schwann cells of NF. The spindle cells can be haphazardly arranged in a myxoid or densely collagenous stroma, with compact bundles of collagen-rich cytoplasmic processes and stroma, akin to the "shredded carrots" appearance common in NF. In others, spindle cells are organized in parallel or "stacked" arrangements. Fascicular growth may be evident (Figs. 4.25 and 4.26).

Fig. 4.4 Solitary neurofibroma: the proliferation may be highly collagenous and blend imperceptibly with the adjacent dermis

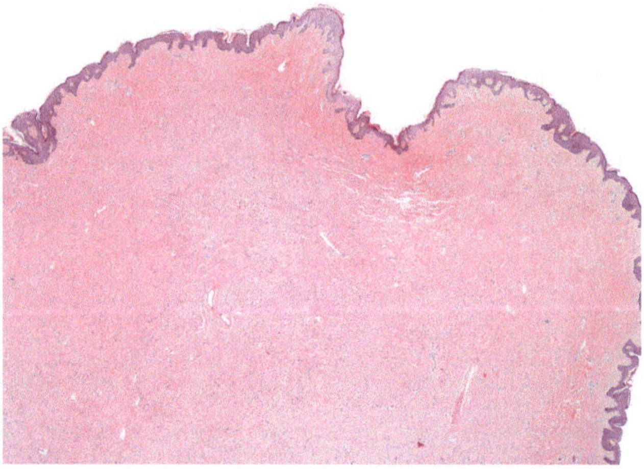

Fig. 4.5 Solitary neurofibroma: lesions are commonly pedunculated or polypoid

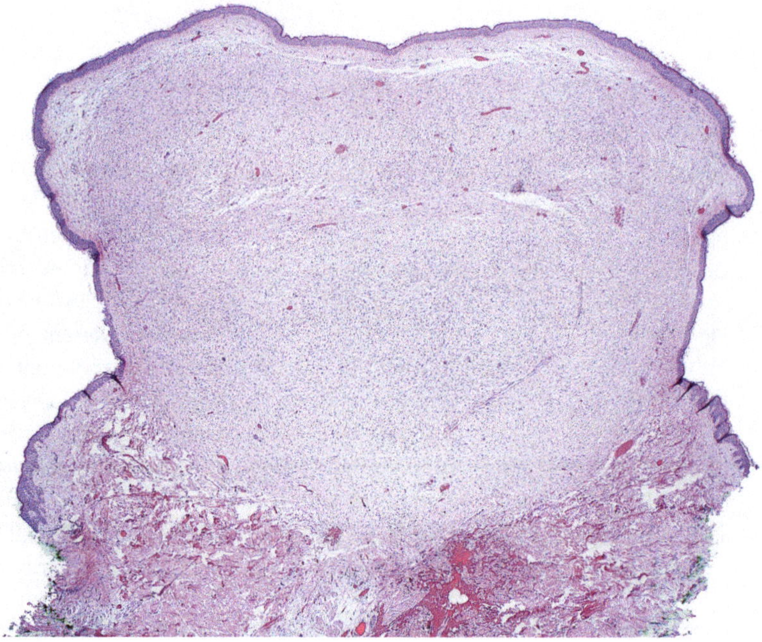

Fig. 4.6 Neurofibroma: the lesional cells consist mainly of Schwann cells with uniform ovoid to spindled nuclei. The cells have finely fibrillar cytoplasm and the background is pale and eosinophilic. Small blood vessels are often prominent

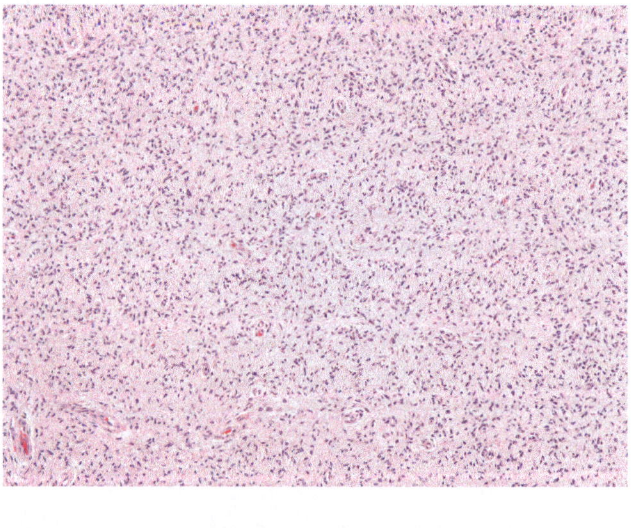

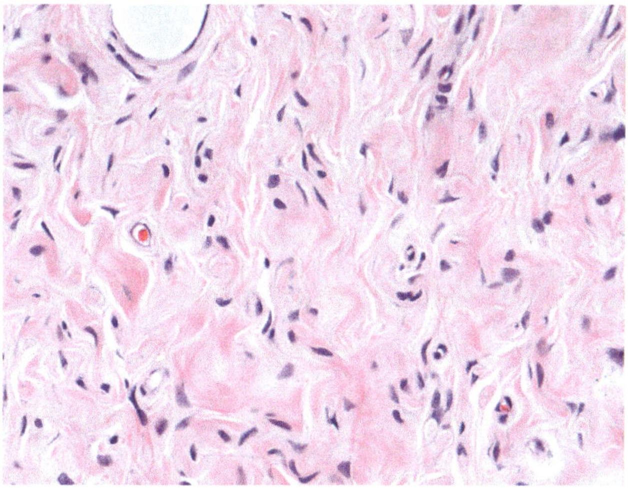

Fig. 4.7 Neurofibroma: the Schwann cells have delicate fibrillar cytoplasmic processes. Their arrangement is seemingly haphazard. Polygonal stromal cells are admixed

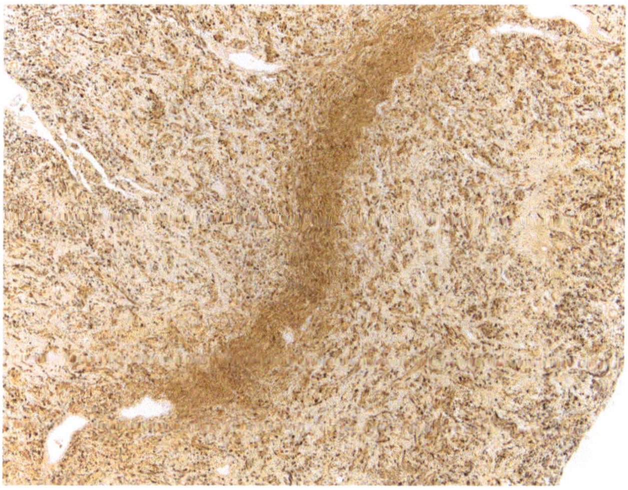

Fig. 4.8 S-100 protein expression in *neurofibroma*: the majority, but not all cells express this marker. A residual portion of the nerve is present centrally

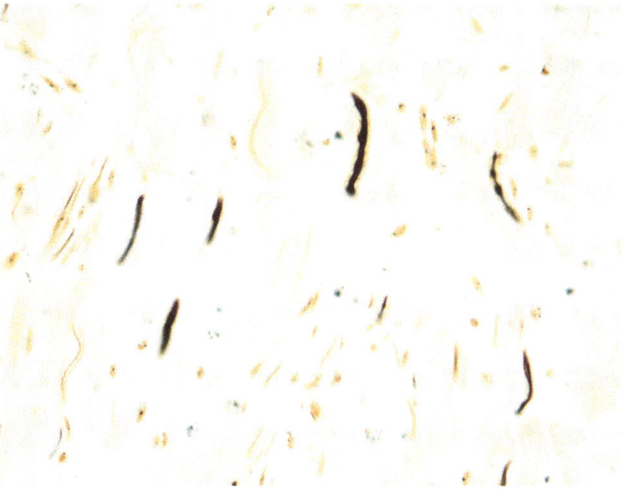

Fig. 4.9 Bielschowsky stain highlights many axons (*dark brown-black*) in neurofibroma. This silver-containing histochemical stain has been largely replaced by immunohistochemical methods

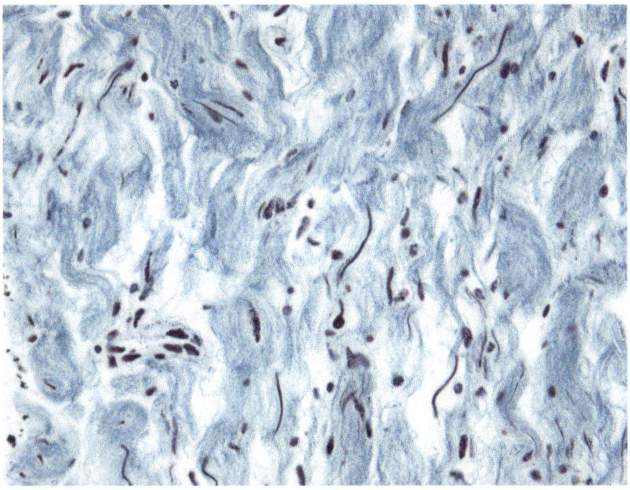

Fig. 4.10 Bodian stain: silver also highlights axons (*black*)

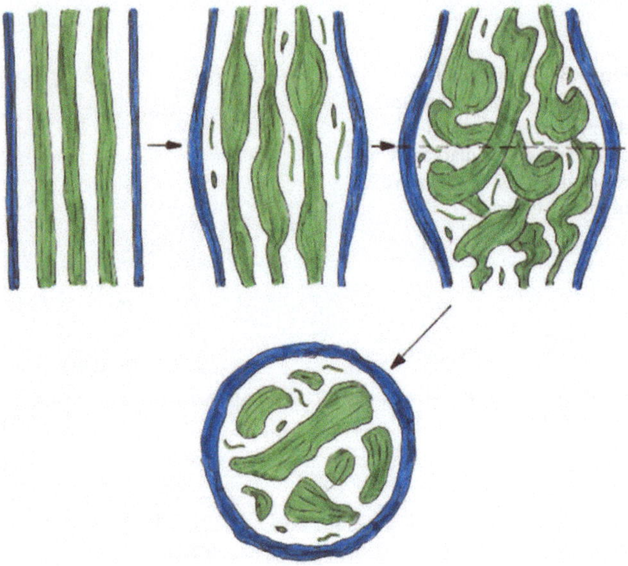

Fig. 4.11 Schematic drawing of *plexiform neurofibroma*: conceptually there is an expansion of large fascicles within the parent nerve. Larger fascicles are present in the soft tissue or deep subcutis accounting for the location of plexiform variants. These forms do not arise primarily in the dermis but may extend into the dermis secondarily. When cut in perpendicular planes these appear as multiple separate nodules (artwork by ZA)

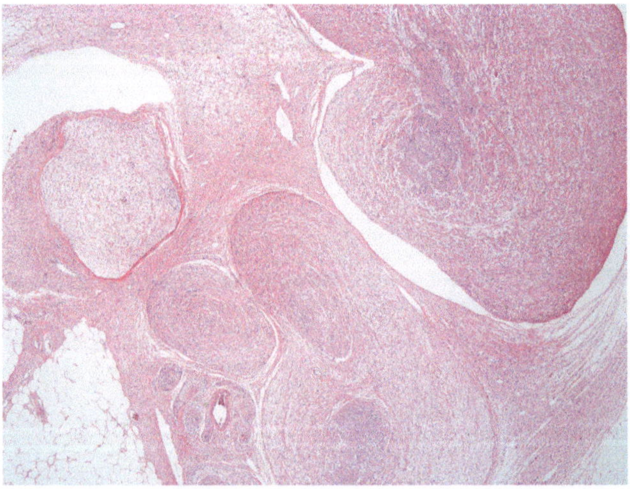

Fig. 4.12 Plexiform neurofibroma: multiple nodules are present. Both the nodules and intervening areas are composed of neurofibroma. There are variable amounts of myxoid stroma and densely collagenous areas, common to this entity

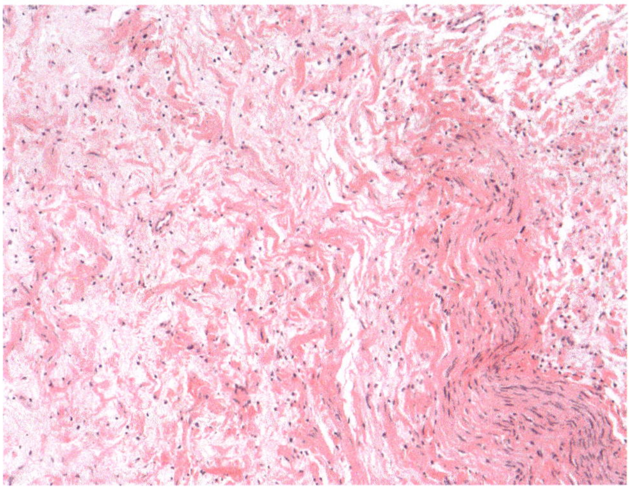

Fig. 4.13 Neurofibroma: compact bundles of collagen-rich stroma and cytoplasmic processes emanating from the Schwann cells resemble "shredded carrots." This finding is more common in subcutaneous forms. Note the presence of residual nerve fascicle (*right*)

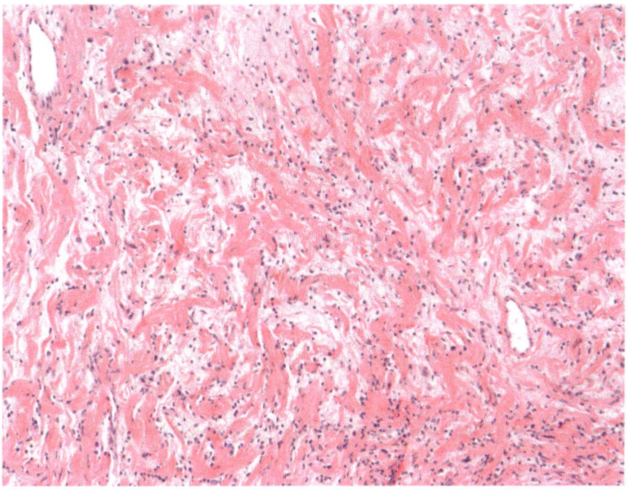

Fig. 4.14 Neurofibroma: compact bundles of collagen-rich stroma and cytoplasmic processes emanating from the Schwann cells resemble "shredded carrots." This finding is more common in subcutaneous forms (higher magnification)

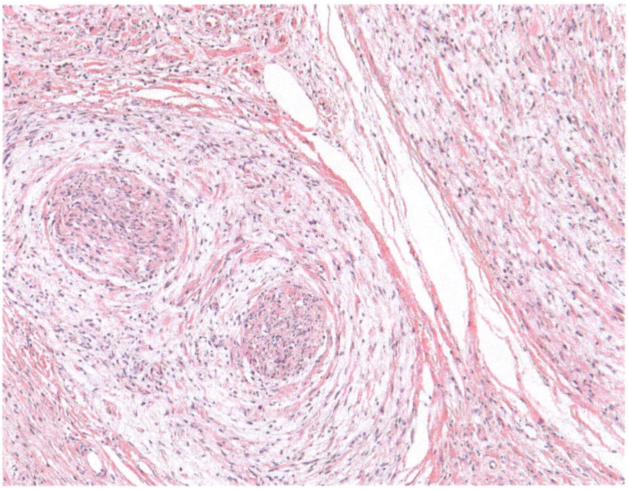

Fig. 4.15 Neurofibroma: the lesion surrounds two residual nerve fascicles. This illustrates how neurofibroma arises from within the nerve fascicle and includes each of the normal constituents of the fascicle including some of the normal fibers and fascicles

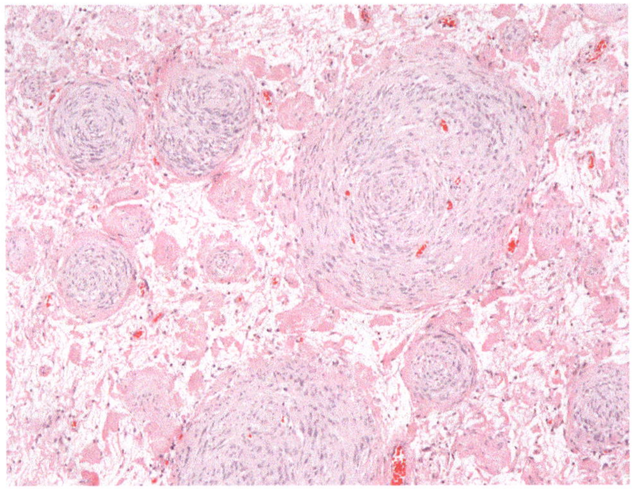

Fig. 4.16 Schwann cell nodules in neurofibroma: occasionally foci rich in Schwann cells may be present, mimicking either residual nerve or schwannoma

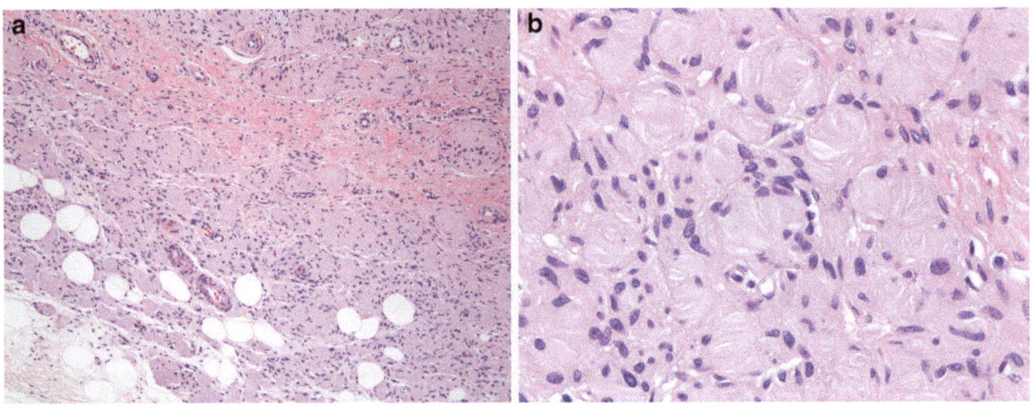

Fig. 4.17 (**a**, **b**) Pseudomeissnerian bodies in neurofibroma: rounded collections of Schwann cells and collagen resemble Meissner corpuscles

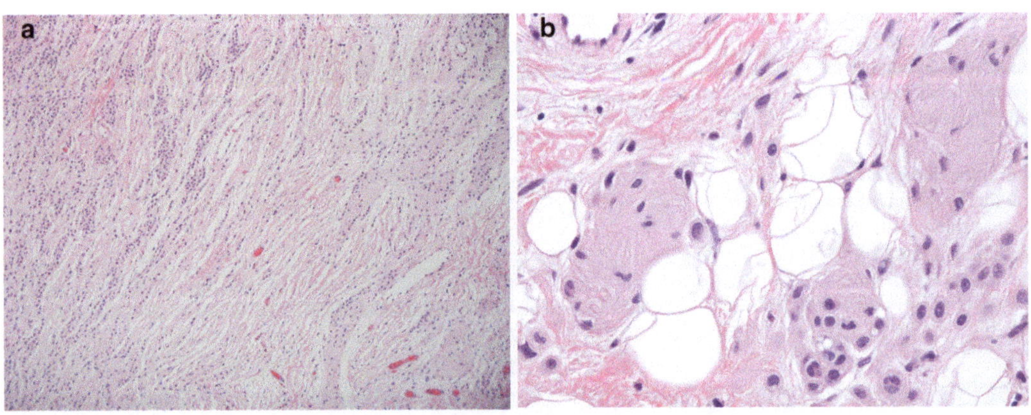

Fig. 4.18 Melanocytic nevi with "neurotization": (**a**) slender spindled melanocytic nevus cells (*right*) resemble those of neurofibroma. Typical epithelioid nevus cells are present (*left*) allowing for distinction from a true neural lesion. (**b**) Pseudomeissnerian bodies in an intradermal nevus resemble those of neurofibroma

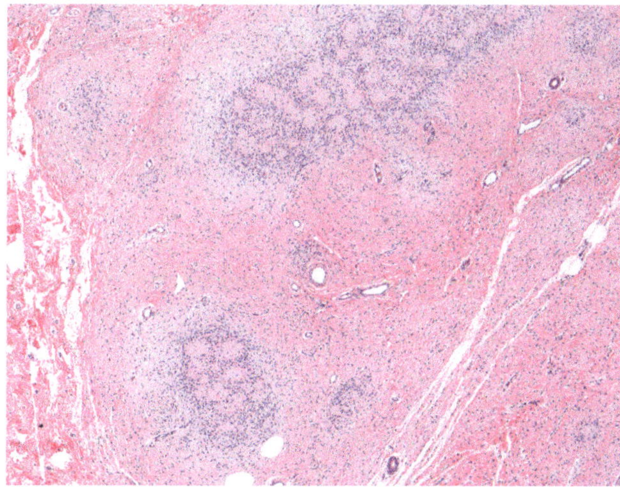

Fig. 4.19 Dendritic cell neurofibroma with pseudorosettes: sharply delineated nodules (top and bottom center) with rosette-like structure are present in a background otherwise typical of neurofibroma

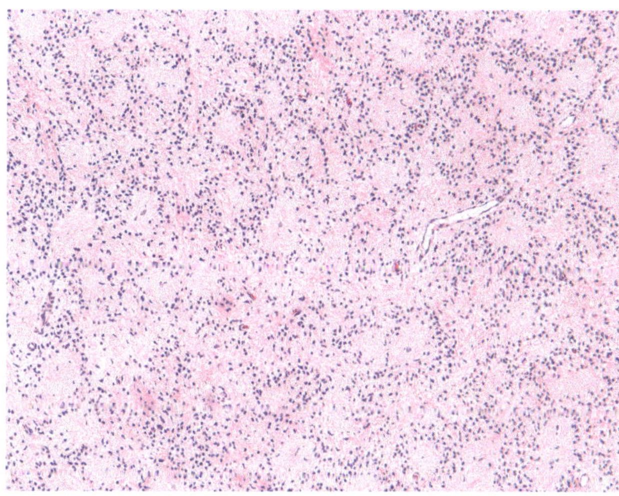

Fig. 4.20 Dendritic cell neurofibroma with pseudorosettes: Schwann cell nuclei align peripheral to aggregates of cytoplasmic extensions resembling Homer Wright rosettes. Cells with large nuclei are identified in the center of some of the structures

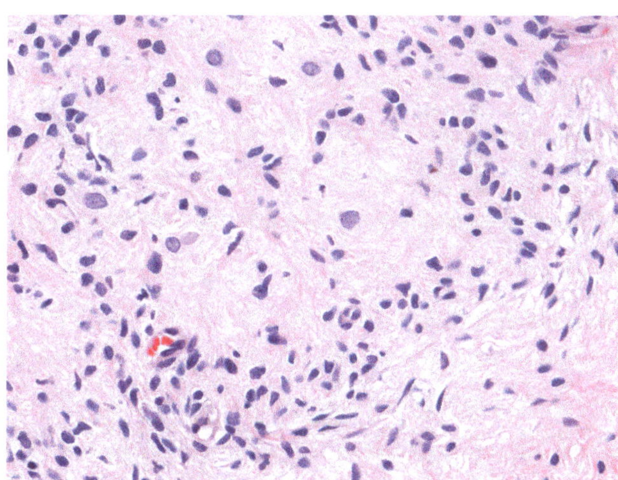

Fig. 4.21 Dendritic cell neurofibroma with pseudorosettes: cells with a prominent polygonal nucleus and fine chromatin are present in the center of some rosettes. These have prominent dendritic processes best visualized by S-100 protein immunostain

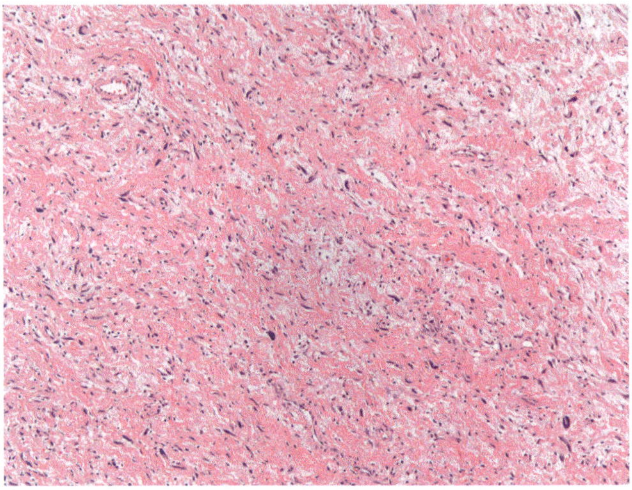

Fig. 4.22 Atypical neurofibroma: scattered cells have dark, large, and irregular nuclei. The background of dense collagen-rich bundles ("shredded carrots") and myxoid changes is characteristic of neurofibroma

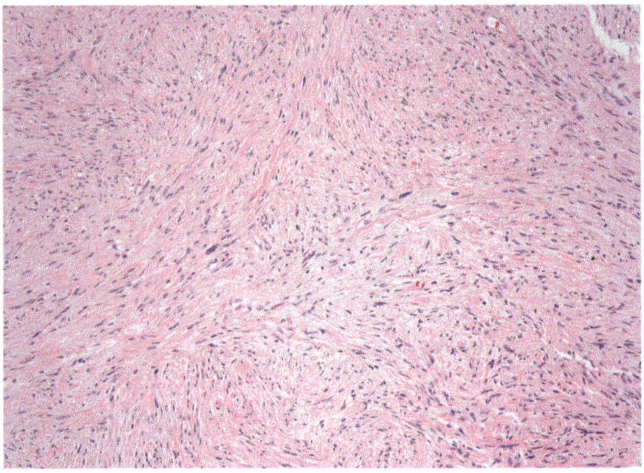

Fig. 4.23 Atypical neurofibroma: this variant is composed of atypical cells arranged in intersecting fascicles. The atypical cells are widely spaced and lack mitotic activity, features distinguishing this lesion from malignant peripheral nerve sheath tumor

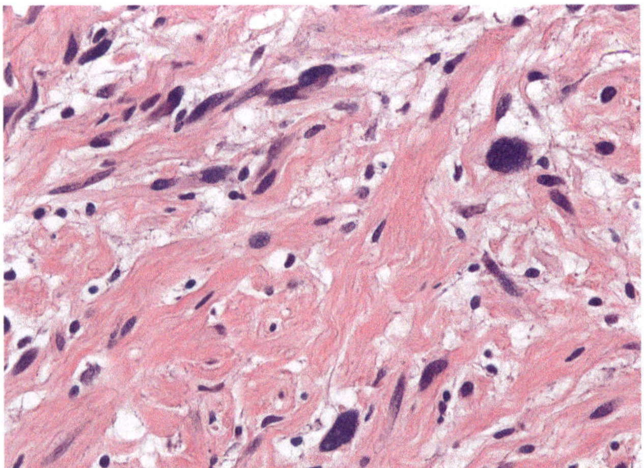

Fig. 4.24 Atypical neurofibroma: some nuclei are highly pleomorphic. These are hyperchromatic with smudgy chromatin, similar to those of ancient schwannoma. These cells are positive for S-100 protein and type IV collagen, and share ultrastructural features of Schwann cells

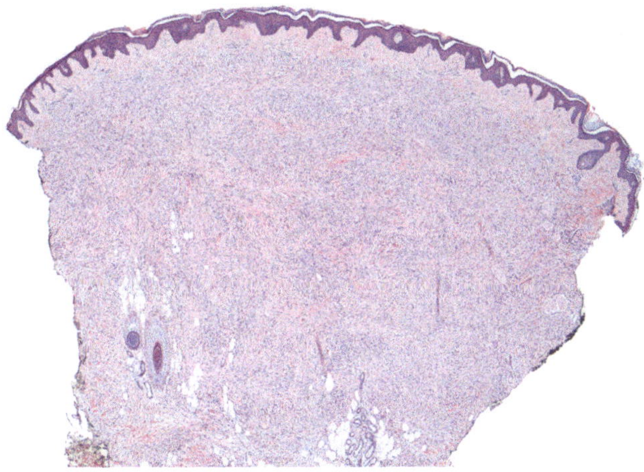

Fig. 4.25 Cellular neurofibroma: a spindle cell proliferation involves the entire dermis but is separated from the epidermis by a Grenz zone

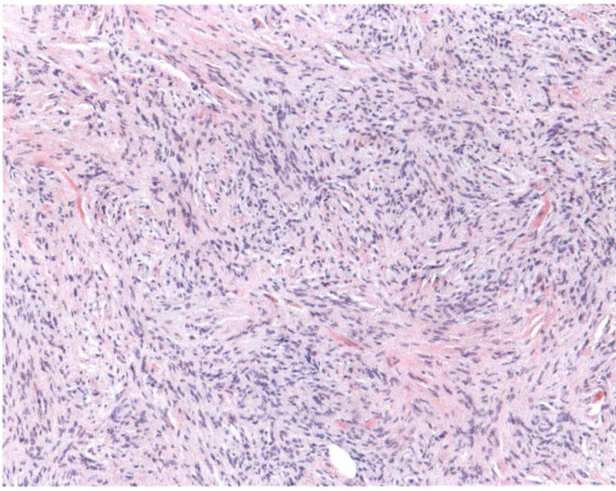

Fig. 4.26 Cellular neurofibroma: increased density of spindle cells otherwise characteristic of the Schwann cells in ordinary neurofibroma. There is a finely fibrillar appearance, also characteristic of neurofibroma. This should be distinguished from spindle cell melanoma. Lack of mitotic activity, pleomorphism, and necrosis distinguish this from malignant peripheral nerve sheath tumor

Cellularity may be increased so that focal cell–cell contacts are present. Dense cellularity with marked nuclear crowding with exclusion of intervening stroma is not seen; if present, MPNST should be considered.

Pigmented NF is an unusual variant of NF, composed of the typical mixture of Schwann cells, perineurial cells, and fibrocytes, in addition to a population of melanin-laden cells (Fig. 4.27). The pigmented cells may have a spindled, dendritic, or less often, epithelioid appearance (Fig. 4.28). The pigmented cells express S-100 protein and melanocytic markers such as Melan-A indicating a melanocytic phenotype. The pigment is highlighted by Fontana-Masson stain (Fig. 4.29). It is uncertain whether these are true melanocytes or Schwann cells with melanocytic differentiation, as both arise from the neural crest. Iron stains are negative. Pigmented NF may or may not be associated with NF1.

Myxoid NF is a variant of NF with abundant mucin. Pools of mucin may separate the spindle cells and collagen fibers (Fig. 4.30a, b). A parent nerve of origin may be evident, greatly expanded by the proliferation and myxoid material (Fig. 4.31a, b). Vacuolated histiocytes sometimes termed muciphages or "pseudolipoblasts" may be present.

Epithelioid NF is a rare variant. Some authors describe tumors with this morphology as "benign epithelioid peripheral nerve sheath tumor" as separation from schwannoma may be difficult or even artificial. The term is retained in this work for nerve

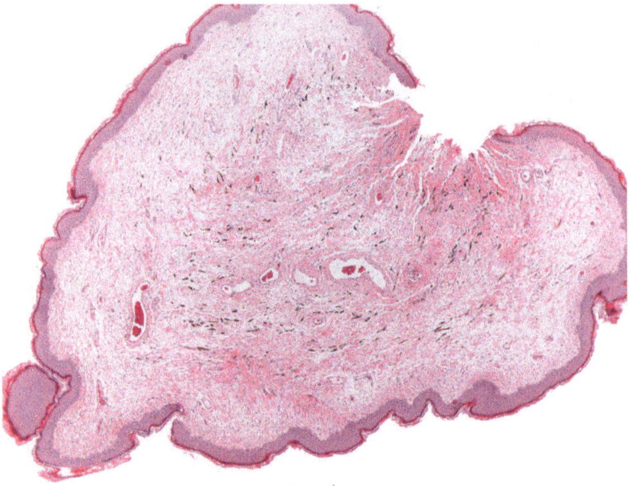

Fig. 4.27 Pigmented neurofibroma: an otherwise typical solitary neurofibroma with scattered pigmented cells

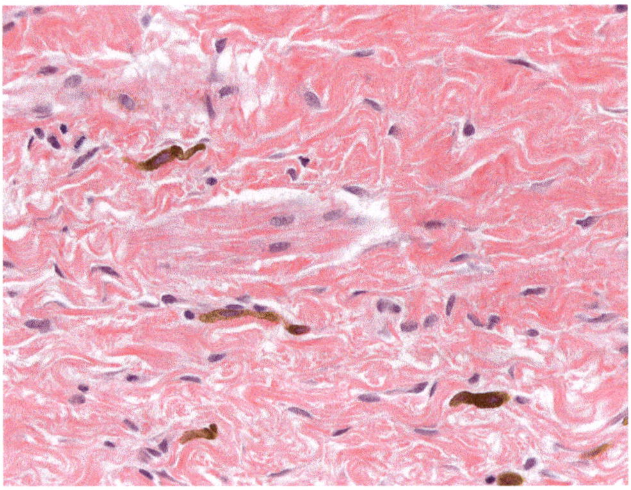

Fig. 4.28 Pigmented neurofibroma: plump golden brown cells are admixed with typical cells and stroma of neurofibroma. The etiology of these cells is uncertain, but these may represent melanocytic differentiation of Schwann cells

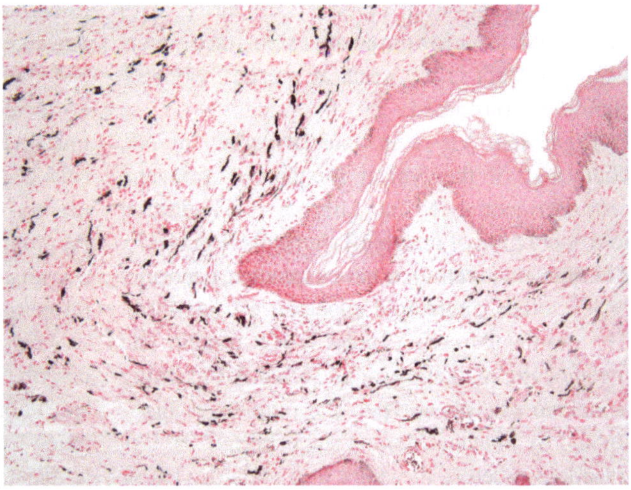

Fig. 4.29 Pigmented neurofibroma: Fontana-Masson stain confirms the presence of melanin

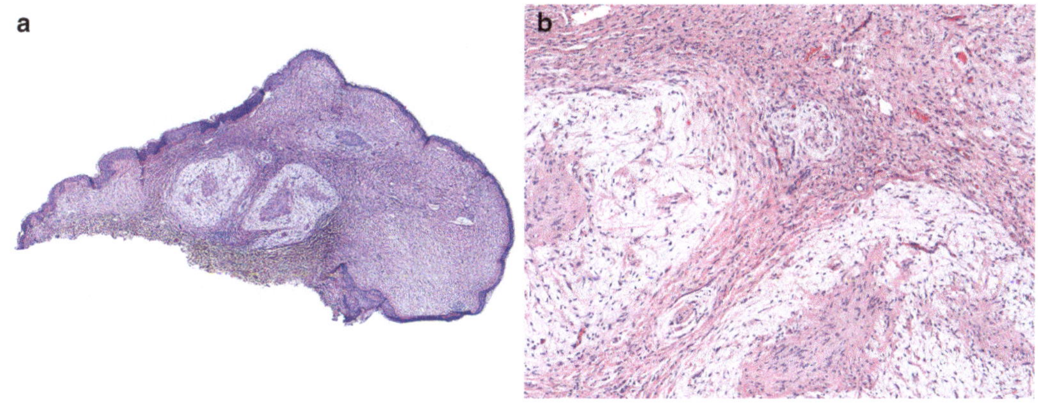

Fig. 4.30 Myxoid neurofibroma: (**a**) mucopolysaccharides may accumulate in well-delineated nodules within the tumor. (**b**) In some cases, the Schwann cells in these cellular foci may resemble Verocay bodies. The haphazard proliferation around the nodules and lack of a capsule is typical of neurofibroma and distinguishes it from schwannoma

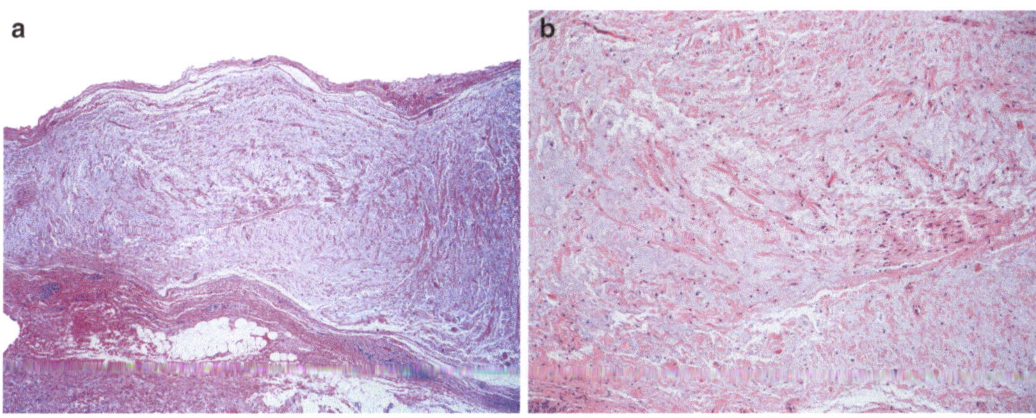

Fig. 4.31 Myxoid neurofibroma: (**a**) at low power the general outline of a nerve is visible. This patient has type 1 neurofibromatosis. (**b**) Most of the nerve is replaced by myxoid material and collagen-rich Schwann cells arranged in short bundles. Residual nerve is visible (*right center*)

sheath proliferations that contain axons and lack a defined capsule, features otherwise used for the separation of schwannoma and neurofibroma (Fig. 4.32). Epithelioid NF is composed of cells with round to slightly irregular nuclei, and often with degenerative type changes including intranuclear pseudoinclusions. Cytoplasm is eosinophilic and abundant although often poorly defined (Fig. 4.33). Binucleate and multinucleated cells are present. The stroma may be myxoid or vaguely chondroid, but in many cases the stroma is heavily collagenous.

Perineurioma-like NF is a tumor with overlapping features of NF and perineurioma. These "hybrid" tumors are composed of Schwann cells with a collagenous background, in addition to EMA-positive cells arranged in cellular whorls like those of perineurioma (Fig. 4.34). A retained background typical of NF is present. A subset of atypical NF with a lamellar growth pattern also show overlapping histologic and immunohistochemical features of perineurial differentiation.

Lipomatous NF is an uncommon histologic variant defined by the presence of admixed adipocytes (Fig. 4.35). Typical features of NF, namely, a bland spindle cell proliferation set in a variably collagenous fibrillar background, are present (Fig. 4.36). Similar tumors with cells resembling lipoblasts have been described as *lipoblastic nerve sheath tumors*. Both the Schwann cells and adipocytes express S-100 protein (Fig. 4.37).

Differential Diagnosis

Common solitary neurofibroma is distinguished from schwannoma by the lack of a thick collagenous capsule and its heterogeneous appearance. Schwannoma on the other hand is composed chiefly of Schwann cells. Although only a portion of cells in NF expresses S-100 protein, schwannoma is diffusely positive. Axons are more abundant in NF but absent or only rarely present at the periphery of schwannoma. NF lacks Verocay body formation in most cases, although in some there are nodules of Schwann cells that can form these structures. Distinction from a heavily "neurotized" intradermal or combined melanocytic nevus may be difficult. The presence of type A or B epithelioid nevus cells, prominent extension along adnexal structures and if necessary, immunohistochemistry (i.e., Melan-A stain) should lead to the correct diagnosis. Of great importance is excluding a desmoplastic or neurotropic melanoma with extreme schwannian differentiation, especially in those NF with atypical cells or increased cellularity. Melanoma should especially be considered in the setting of marked solar elastosis. The cytologic appearance of the cells may be identical,

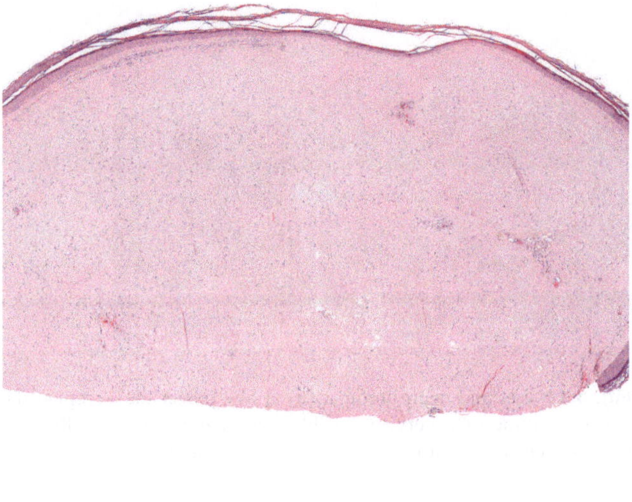

Fig. 4.32 Epithelioid neurofibroma: a circumscribed nodular proliferation involves nearly the entire dermis except for a small Grenz zone. The stroma is densely collagenous, resembling sclerotic fibroma

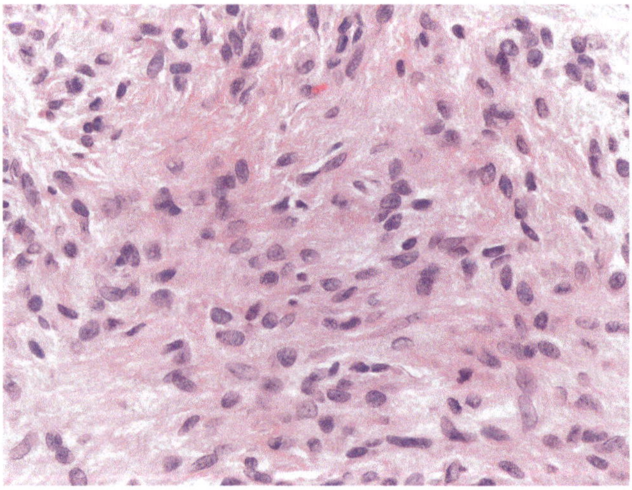

Fig. 4.33 Epithelioid neurofibroma: in this example the lesional cells have plump nuclei with uniform chromatin and a fine fibrillar cytoplasm

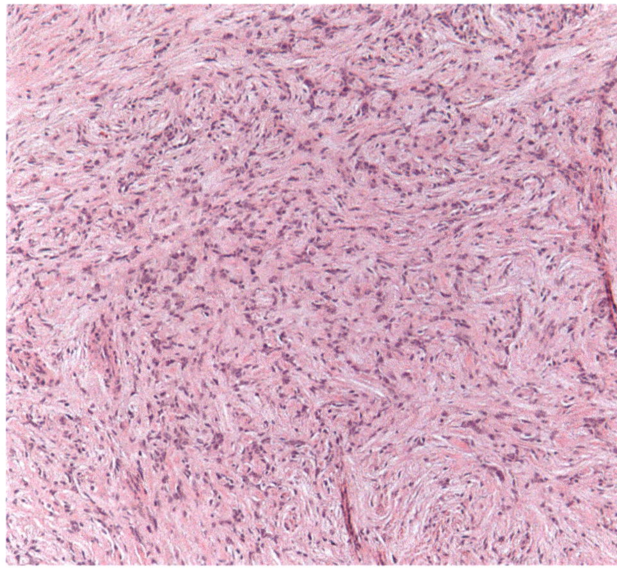

Fig. 4.34 Neurofibroma with perineurioma-like features: epithelioid cells in thin cords and trabeculae are surrounded by spindle cells. By immunohistochemistry the spindle cells are positive for S-100 protein while the epithelioid cells express EMA

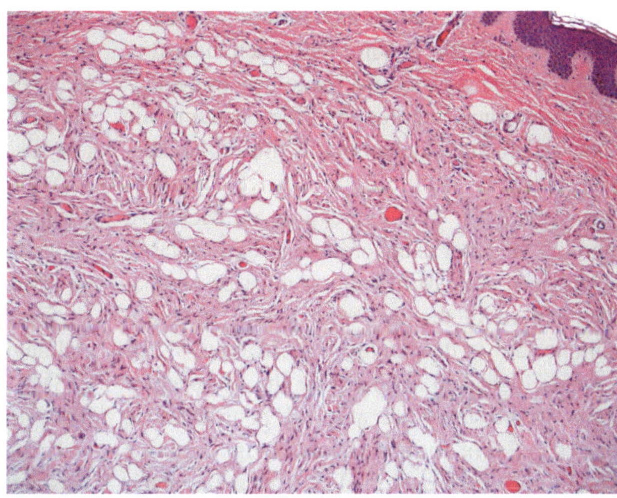

Fig. 4.35 Lipomatous neurofibroma: a circumscribed proliferation of spindle cells with admixed adipocytes

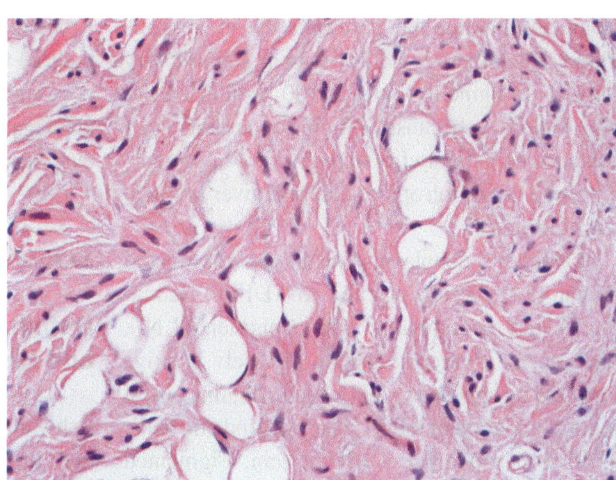

Fig. 4.36 Lipomatous neurofibroma: the spindle cells have fibrillar cytoplasm typical of neurofibroma. Adipocytes have thin compressed nuclei at the periphery of the cell

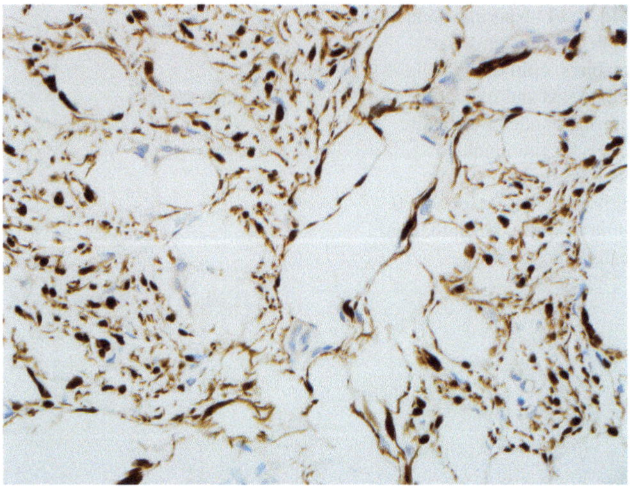

Fig. 4.37 Lipomatous neurofibroma: S-100 protein immunostain highlights both the Schwann cells and adipocytes

although by extensive sampling the more characteristic infiltrative pattern and variation of dense and hypocellular areas commonly seen in desmoplastic melanomas usually becomes more evident. Additional features favoring desmoplastic melanoma include melanoma in situ in the adjacent epidermis, mitotic figures, patchy lymphocyte aggregates, and expression of Melan-A, although the latter is uncommon in desmoplastic melanomas. A word of caution must be emphasized regarding the use of a neural filaments immunostain in desmoplastic melanoma. While it seems logical to assume that the presence of axons would favor an atypical neurofibroma, small bundles of entrapped nerve twigs are often present in desmoplastic melanomas as the melanoma disintegrates nerve twigs into individual axons, mimicking the pattern seen in neurofibroma. Nevertheless, neurofilament stain is very useful in conjunction with S-100 protein and/or with Melan-A, because a high concentration of cells around nerve twigs strongly favor perineurial spread or neurotropic melanoma over atypical neurofibroma.

Nonneural neoplasms such as pigmented dermatofibrosarcoma protuberans (DFSP; Bednar tumor) may occasionally mimic pigmented NF; however, the former is usually diffusely positive for CD34 as opposed to NF, which contains only a minor population of CD34 positive dendritic cells. DFSP is negative for S-100 protein. Pigmented (melanotic) schwannoma can also resemble the pigmented form of NF and may be indistinguishable in some cases. A characteristic myxoid and collagenous background of NF without fascicle or Verocay body formation favors NF. A combined nevus composed of blue nevus and acquired nevus may also resemble pigmented NF.

Myxoid NF has features otherwise diagnostic of NF, leading to ready diagnosis. Awareness of potentially abundant myxoid stroma in NF is important; however, as partial sampling of the tumor may lead to consideration of cutaneous mucinosis, superficial angiomyxoma, dermal nerve sheath myxoma (NSM), myxoid forms of neurothekeoma, and low-grade myxofibrosarcoma.

Epithelioid NF is distinguished from epithelioid schwannoma by the presence of axons in central areas of the mass, and lack of well-defined capsule. Epithelioid NF should be distinguished from epithelioid fibrous histiocytoma, solitary reticulohistiocytoma, and cellular neurothekeoma, all of which are negative for S-100 protein. Intradermal melanocytic nevus is positive for Melan-A.

Schwannoma

Definition, Classification, and Histogenesis

Schwannoma is a benign neoplasm of Schwann cell lineage that like NF, is one of the more frequently encountered cutaneous peripheral nerve sheath tumors. Unlike neurofibroma, schwannoma is composed of an exclusive proliferation of Schwann cells within the confinement of the perineurium (Fig. 4.38a, b; line drawing for histogenesis). Whereas NF is an expansion and possibly hamartomatous of the entire nerve and its constituents, schwannoma is a neoplasm that forms a mass adjacent to the nerve of origin.

Clinical

Cutaneous schwannoma is usually sporadic. Schwannoma however may occur in NF1, but this association is not exclusive and unlike plexiform NF, cutaneous schwannoma is not considered pathognomonic of this condition. Multiple schwannomas of the vestibular nerve may be seen in NF2. Schwannomatosis is a clinically descriptive term that refers to multiple cutaneous schwannomas. An association with NF1 or NF2 is not confirmed.

Histopathology

Schwannoma is a neoplasm composed exclusively of Schwann cells. Like neurofibroma, numerous histopathologic variants of schwannoma are described (Table 4.2).

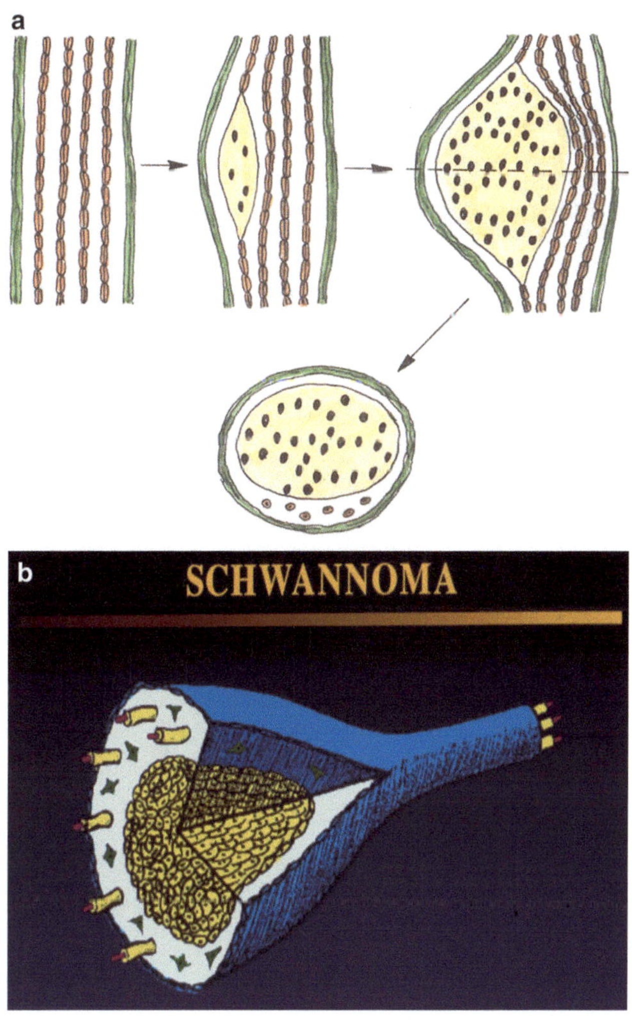

Fig. 4.38 (**a**, **b**) Schematic representation of *schwannoma*: a neoplastic proliferation of Schwann cells arising from a nerve fiber gradually expands the entire fascicle from within, in an eccentric manner, leaving portions of the fascicle uninvolved. The lesion acquires a capsule from the perineurium and surrounding tissue (artwork by ZA)

The usual or common form of schwannoma is a circumscribed mass surrounded by a thick collagenous capsule (Figs. 4.39–4.41). In most forms, there is a variable mixture of hypercellular and hypocellular areas. Hypercellular zones are known as Antoni A areas, and hypocellular areas as Antoni B (Figs. 4.42–4.44). Antoni B areas may have a myxoid or edematous stroma and are by definition Schwann cell-poor. Microcystic changes may be present (Fig. 4.45). The spindle cells stain strongly positive for S-100 protein (Fig. 4.46). Unlike neurofibroma, axons are usually not evident. When present, they are few in number, and are often located at the periphery of the capsule which corresponds to the nerve of origin, rather than diffusely distributed. Small and medium-sized blood vessels are often prominent. In many cases, the vascular walls are thickened and have a hyalinized appearance. In AntoniA areas, the Schwann cell nuclei are

Table 4.2 Schwannoma variants

Common type
Ancient
Cellular
Epithelioid
Pigmented (psammomatous melanotic)
Plexiform cellular
Plexiform
Pseudoglandular

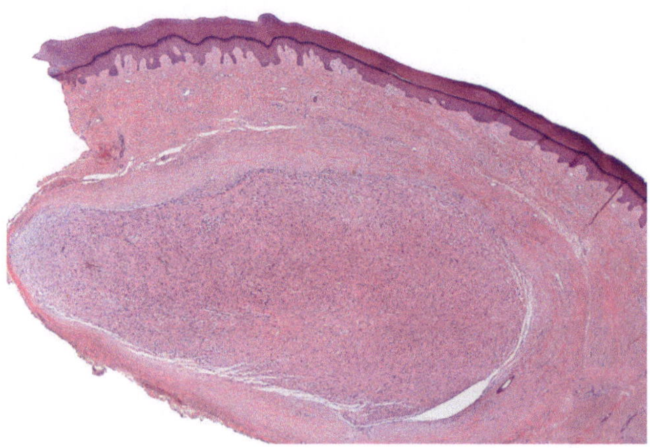

Fig. 4.39 Schwannoma: typical cutaneous forms are encapsulated, circumscribed, and located in the mid-dermis, deep dermis, or subcutis. The capsule is thick and collagenous. Occasional perineurial cells may be present if stained with EMA

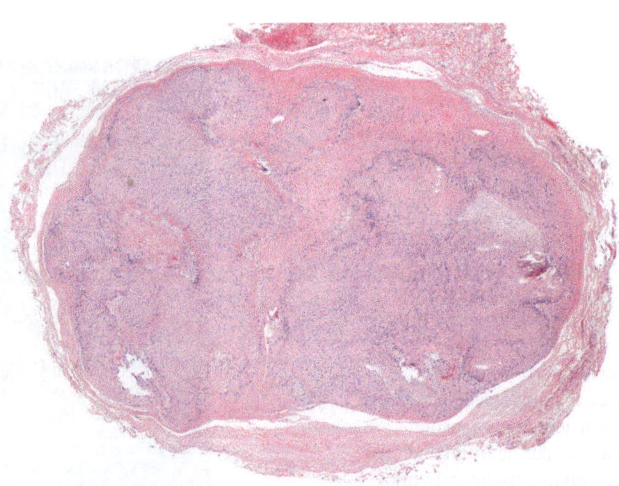

Fig. 4.40 Schwannoma: a subcutaneous form with a mixture of hypercellular (Antoni A) and hypocellular (Antoni B) areas. The latter have collagenous or myxoid stroma, but with few cells

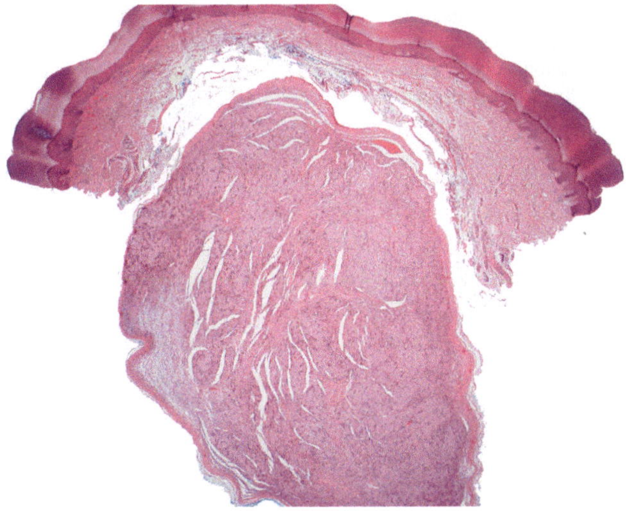

Fig. 4.41 Schwannoma: an encapsulated dermal schwannoma. Artifactual clefts may be present, which can raise consideration of palisaded encapsulated neuroma at first glance

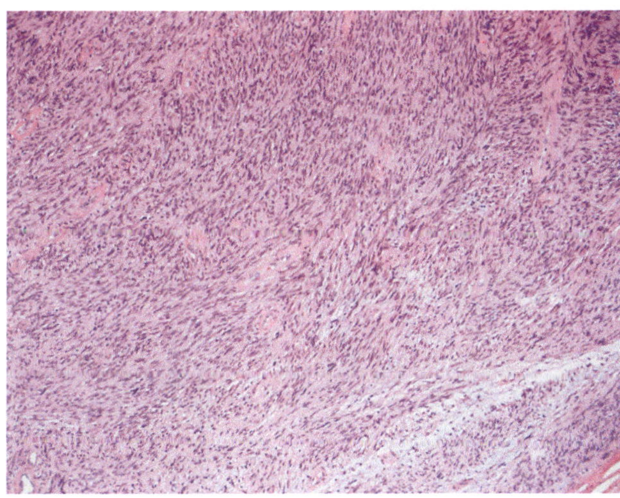

Fig. 4.42 Schwannoma: the neoplastic Schwann cells are arranged in sweeping fascicles. Cellular areas like these are known as Antoni A

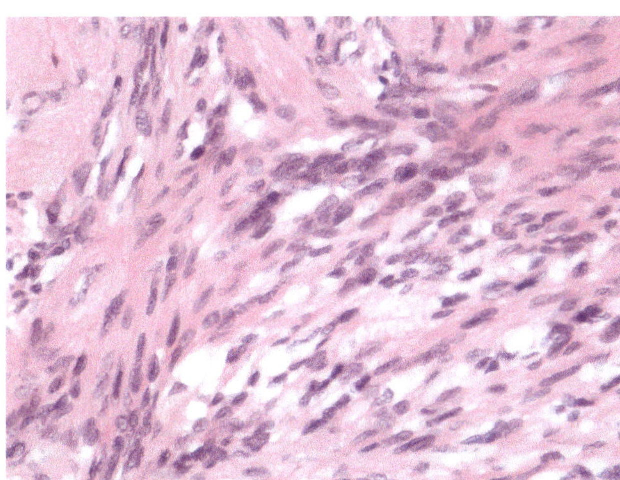

Fig. 4.43 Schwannoma: individual Schwann cells have plump ovoid or slender spindled nuclei with a rounded and a tapered end. Chromatin is often vesicular and intranuclear pseudoinclusions are not uncommon

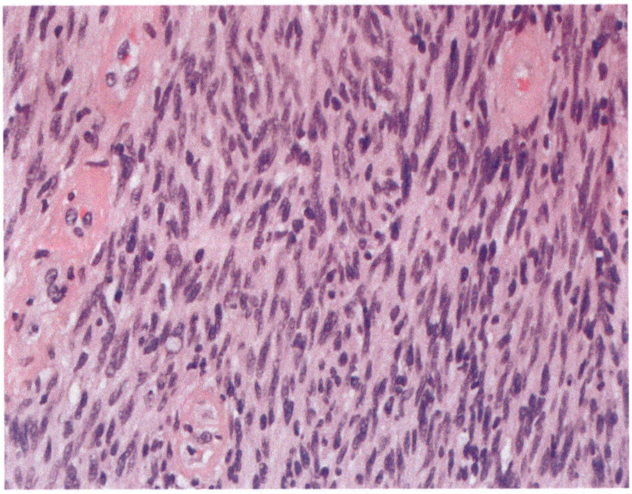

Fig. 4.44 Schwannoma: showing a hypercellular area, Antoni A type, with more hyperchromatic cells

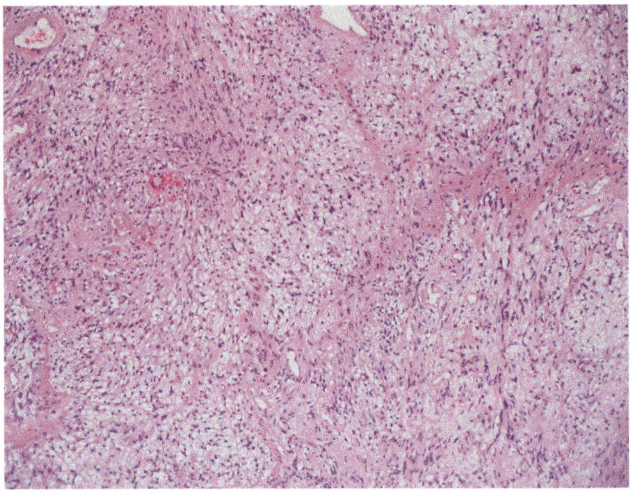

Fig. 4.45 Schwannoma: some forms have a microcystic appearance due to vacuoles adjacent to the neoplastic cells

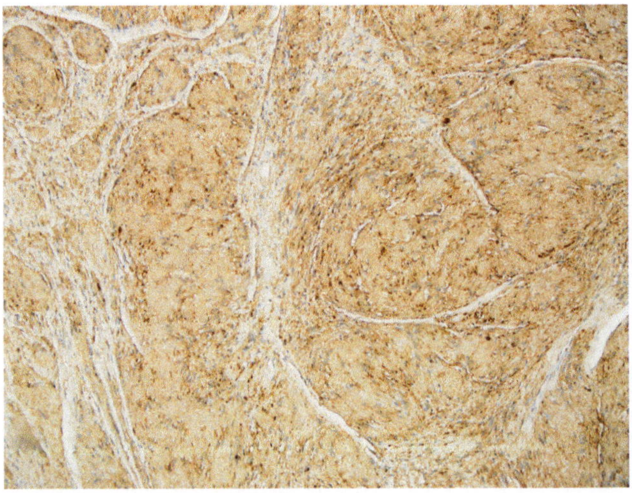

Fig. 4.46 Schwannoma is uniformly positive for S-100 protein

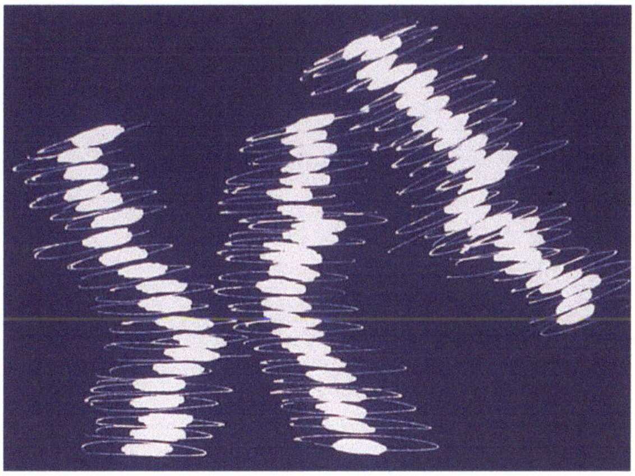

Fig. 4.47 Schematic representation of *nuclear palisading* in schwannoma: nuclei tend to align in parallel arrays like a picket fence (artwork by ZA)

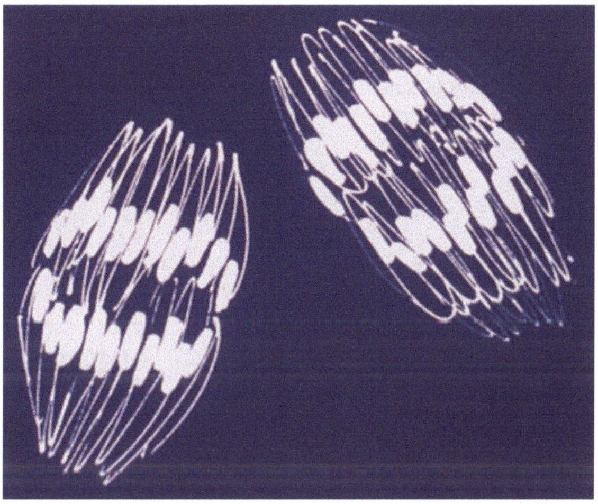

Fig. 4.48 Schematic representation of *Verocay bodies* in schwannoma: nuclear palisades arranged in delineated structures with central areas of collagen-rich cytoplasmic processes and stroma (artwork by ZA)

oriented in fascicles, or aligned in parallel rows known as *nuclear palisading* (Fig. 4.47). In some areas, nuclear palisades are present around a central zone rich in collagen and cytoplasmic processes, but devoid of nuclei resembling "baskets of bananas" (Figs. 4.48–4.53). These structures are referred to as *Verocay bodies*. Similar rounder formations known as collagenous pseudorosettes may also be present. These resemble rosettes found in neuroblastoma, or collagenous spherulosis of the breast or salivary gland (Figs. 4.54 and 4.55).

Ancient schwannoma is a term that refers to conspicuous degenerative changes that occur in long-standing schwannomas (Fig. 4.56). Ancient schwannomas are composed largely of an Antoni B pattern with prominent myxoid change, edema, or stromal hyalinization (Fig. 4.57). Hemorrhage and hemosiderin deposition can be present (Fig. 4.58). Blood vessels are often large and ectatic, with or without thrombotic changes, and may have thickened or hyalinized walls (Fig. 4.59). The above changes are often present in typical schwannomas, although to a lesser extent. The degenerative changes are often associated with variable nuclear atypia manifested by large, irregular nuclei with coarse chromatin and intranuclear pseudoinclusions. Bizarre polygonal nuclei and sometimes multinucleated cells may be present (Fig. 4.60). Mitotic activity is not evident.

Epithelioid schwannoma is a rare variant of schwannoma composed exclusively of small polygonal cells. Spindle cells, Verocay bodies,

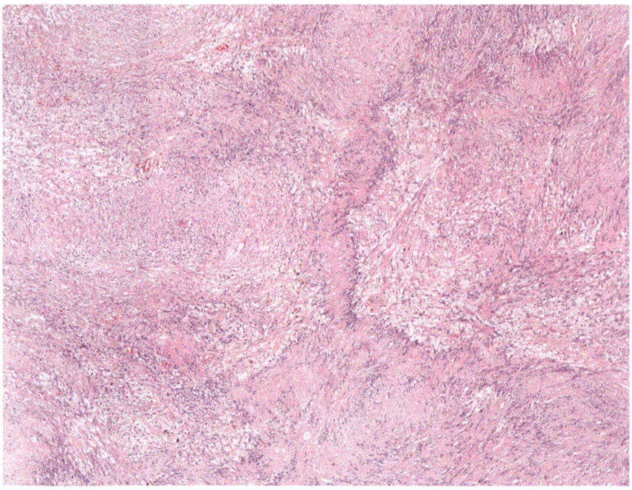

Fig. 4.49 Schwannoma: nuclear palisading

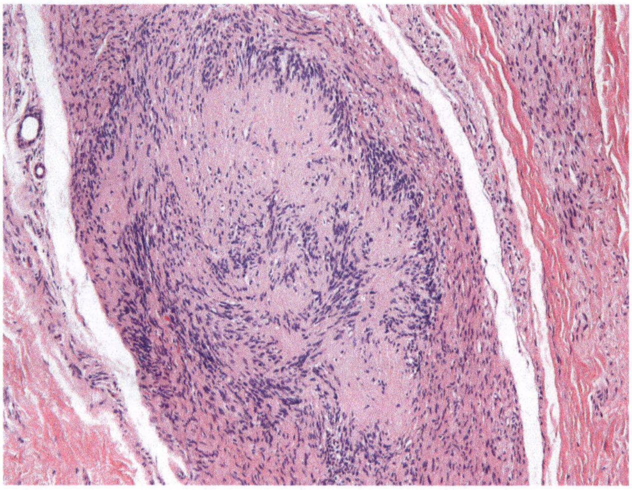

Fig. 4.50 Schwannoma: Verocay body, rounded nodular type

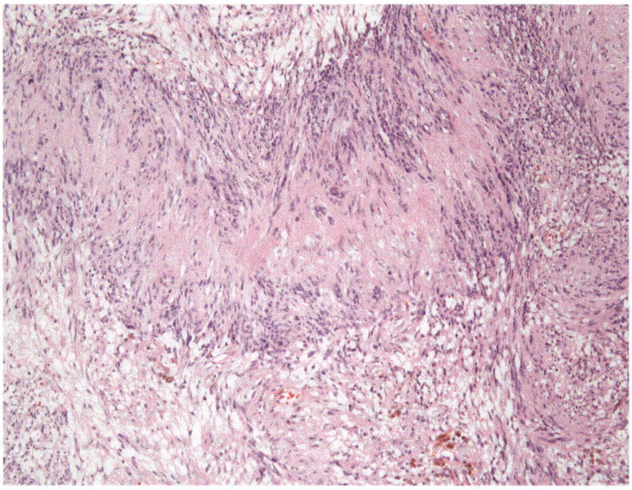

Fig. 4.51 Schwannoma: Verocay body, elongated type. Note the myxoid Antoni B areas *above* and *below*

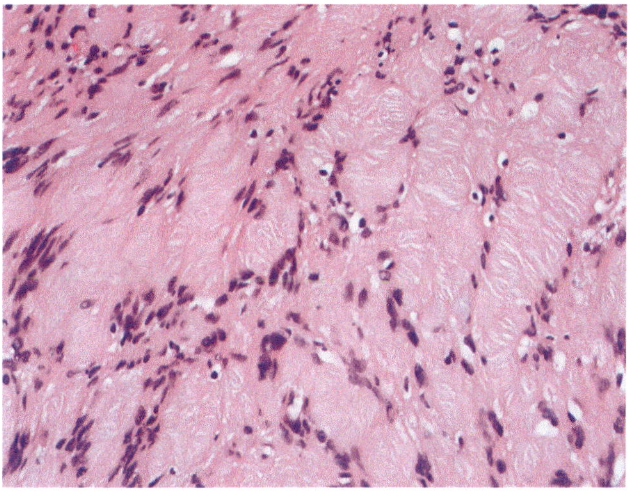

Fig. 4.52 Schwannoma: nuclear palisading may resemble Meissner bodies

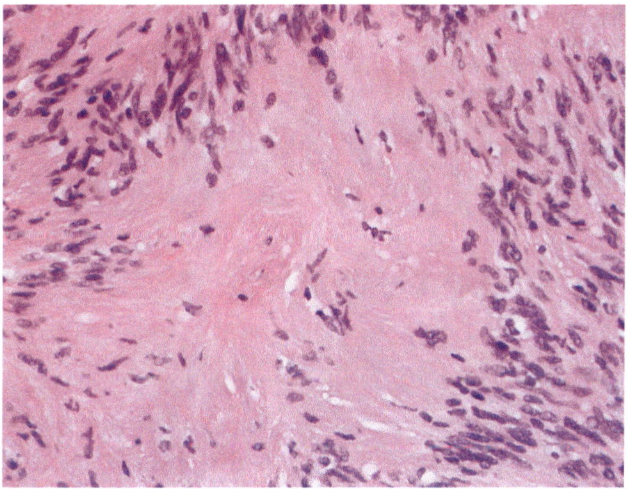

Fig. 4.53 Schwannoma: classical Verocay body

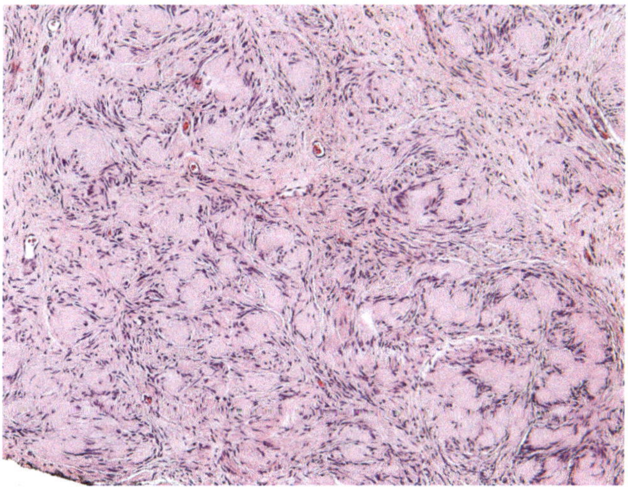

Fig. 4.54 Schwannoma with pseudorosettes: rounded collections of Schwann cells with peripheral nuclear palisading surrounding dense collagenous stroma

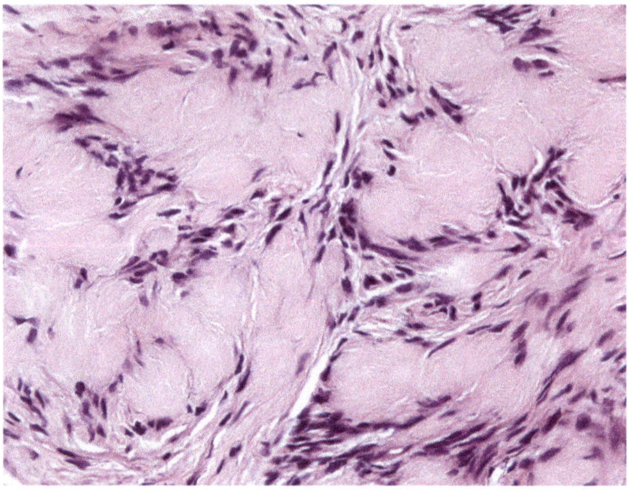

Fig. 4.55 Schwannoma with pseudorosettes: these structures resemble collagenous spherulosis of the breast or salivary gland

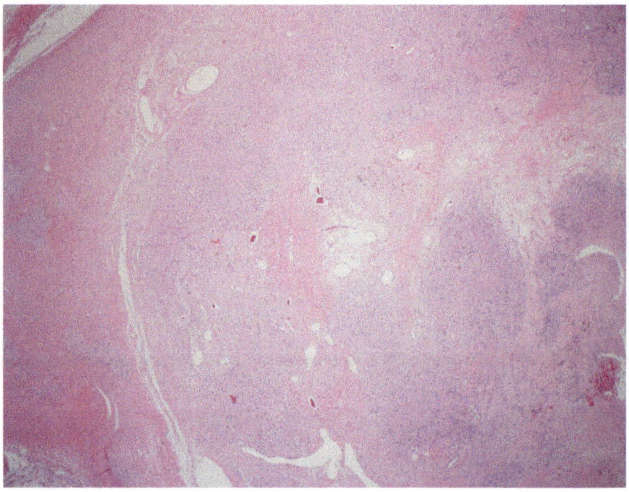

Fig. 4.56 Ancient schwannoma: a mixture of Antoni A and B with large areas of myxoid degeneration. Large vessels are prominent at low magnification

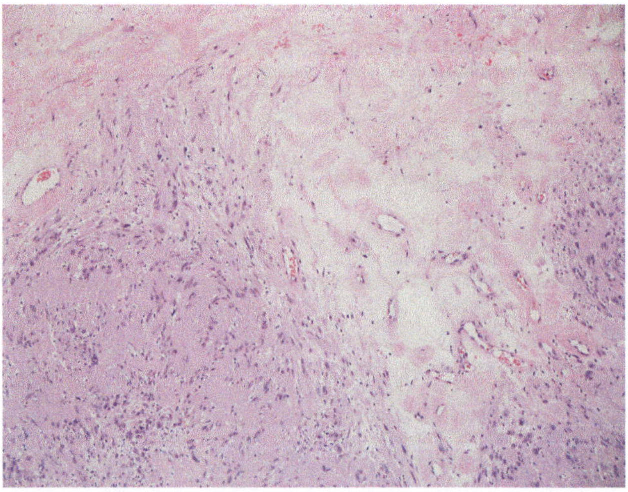

Fig. 4.57 Ancient schwannoma: hypocellular areas with hyalinized vessels adjacent to Antoni A areas with nuclear palisading

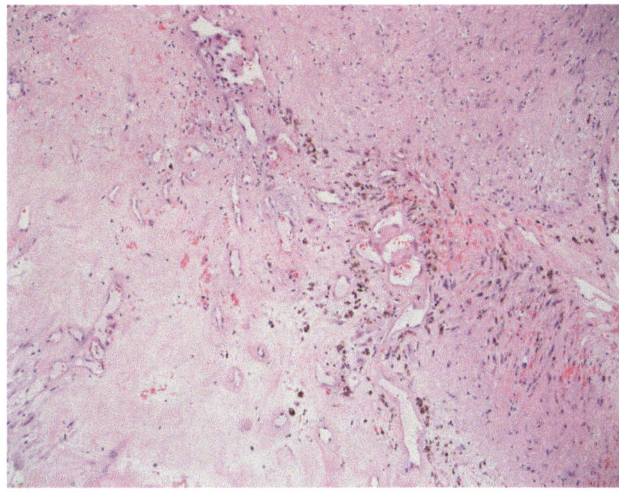

Fig. 4.58 Ancient schwannoma: hemosiderin is present next to the thickened vessels

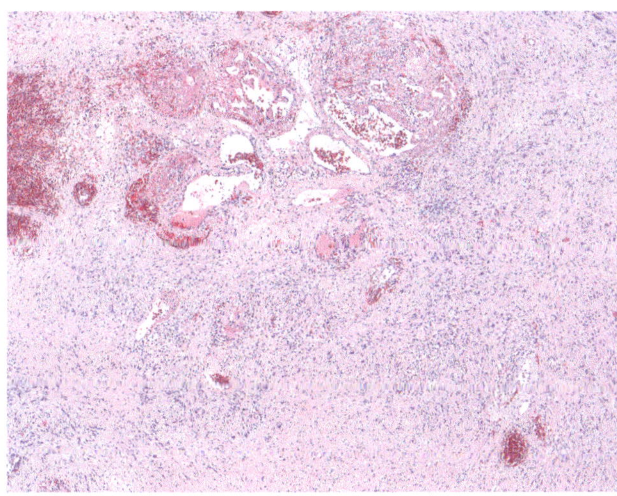

Fig. 4.59 Ancient schwannoma: some vessels are large and ecstatic

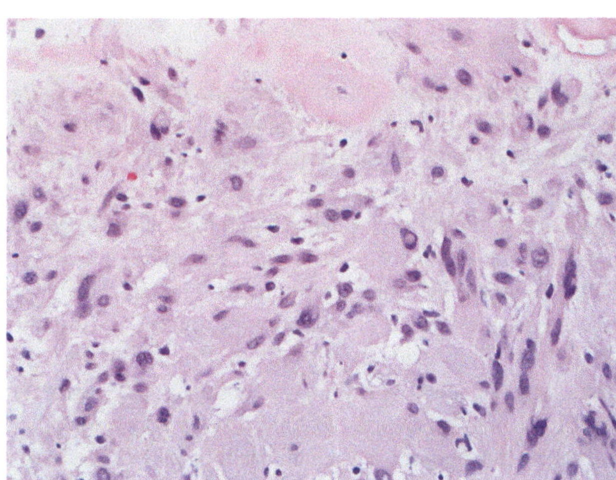

Fig. 4.60 Ancient schwannoma: nuclear atypia is common and likely a degenerative phenomenon. This should not be construed as evidence of malignant change. Many cells have vesicular chromatin and intranuclear cytoplasmic inclusions

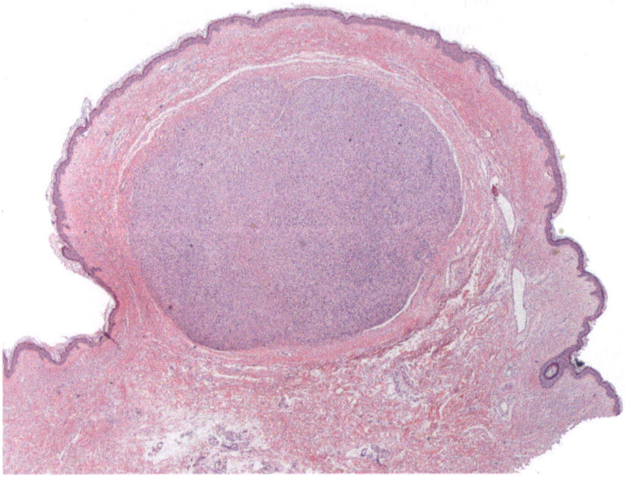

Fig. 4.61 Epithelioid schwannoma: a circumscribed dermal neoplasm with a thick collagenous capsule is also common to this variant

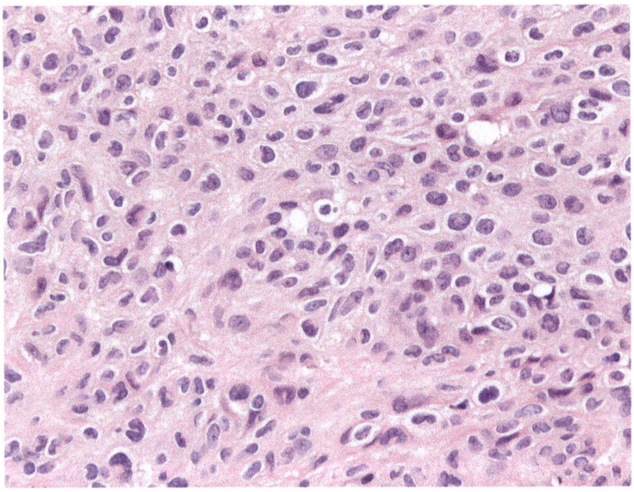

Fig. 4.62 Epithelioid schwannoma: the Schwann cells have round to ovoid nuclei with perinuclear halos. Cell borders may be prominent and resemble nevomelanocytes. The cells are positive for S-100 protein and type IV collagen

and variable cellularity, common in usual types, are absent. These variants are often small, well circumscribed, and encapsulated (Fig. 4.61). The lesional cells have small round nuclei and abundant eosinophilic cytoplasm (Fig. 4.62). The stroma is often densely collagenous and highlighted by type IV collagen immunostain. In some cases, the stroma is exceptionally prominent such that few lesional cells remain. Rosettes reminiscent of neuroblastoma or collagenous spherulosis may be present. Mitotic figures may be present but number less than one per high-power field.

Cellular schwannoma by definition is a schwannoma composed nearly entirely of Antoni A areas (Fig. 4.63). Cellular schwannomas are composed of slightly plump ovoid cells, often larger than the typical spindled Schwann cells of most schwannomas. These however lack obvious pleomorphism and are remarkably monotonous (Fig. 4.64). These are often arranged in fascicles. Verocay bodies may or may not be present. Mitotic figures may be present and although there are no specific data determining the average mitotic activity in cellular schwannoma, some cases may have up to 4 per 10 high-power fields. Focal

Fig. 4.63 Cellular schwannoma: a mass composed solely of hypercellular (Antoni A) growth pattern. The cell density is marked and separation from MPNST is often difficult. Nuclear palisading and Verocay bodies are absent

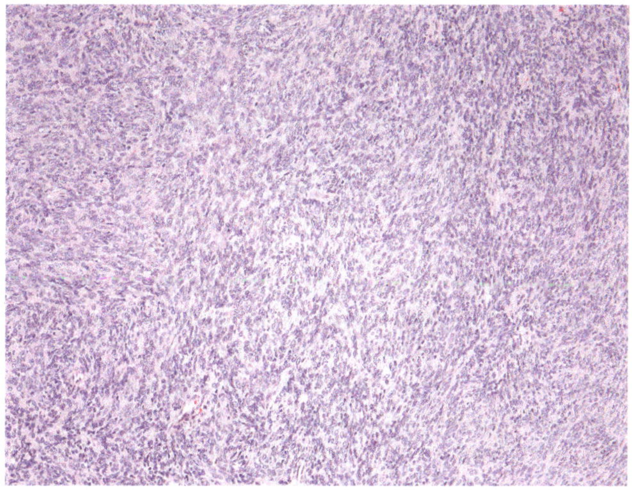

Fig. 4.64 Cellular schwannoma: unlike most MPNST, the nuclei are relatively uniform with vesicular chromatin. This cellular density would not be unusual for cutaneous MPNST and the entire lesion must be evaluated for nuclear pleomorphism, necrosis, and mitotic activity

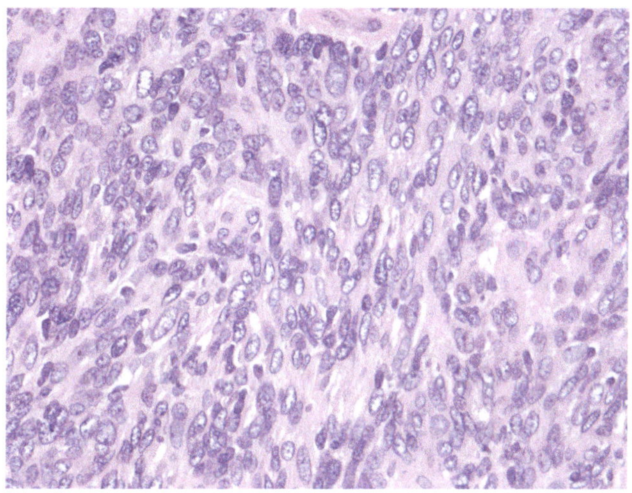

Fig. 4.65 Cellular schwannoma: focal hypocellular areas may be present. In this example, hyalinized blood vessels are also present suggestive of degenerative change

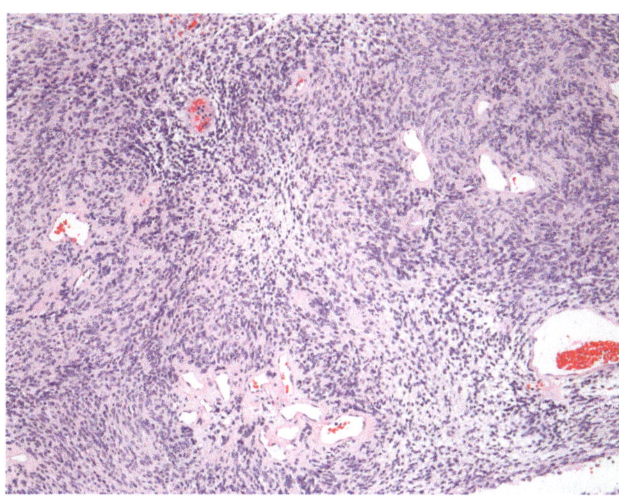

hypocellular areas may be present, but necrosis is absent (Fig. 4.65). This is one of the most diagnostically challenging variants, as it closely resembles melanoma or malignant peripheral nerve sheath tumor.

Plexiform schwannoma, like plexiform neurofibroma, is composed of multiple interconnecting small and large nodules of neoplastic cells (Fig. 4.66). Unlike usual forms of schwannoma, Antoni A areas predominate. Each nodule is encapsulated (Figs. 4.67 and 4.68). There is often mild cytologic atypia manifested as nuclear enlargement, epithelioid change, or polygonal cells. The lesion contains only a few axons as confirmed by immunohistochemical stains to neural filaments. Unlike plexiform neurofibroma, there is no known association with NF1 and no apparent risk of malignant transformation. For more detailed differential diagnostic comparison of plexiform tumors, please refer to Table A.4 in Appendix.

Plexiform cellular schwannoma (congenital neural hamartoma, fascicular schwannoma) is a Schwann cell neoplasm that occurs in infants and may be present at birth. These present as a slightly erythematous plaque or nodule on the trunk or limb. The surface may be covered with hairs. Clinically this may resemble an adnexal or epidermal nevus, or smooth muscle hamartoma. There is a dermal proliferation of multiple small to slightly expanded spindle cell rich fascicles

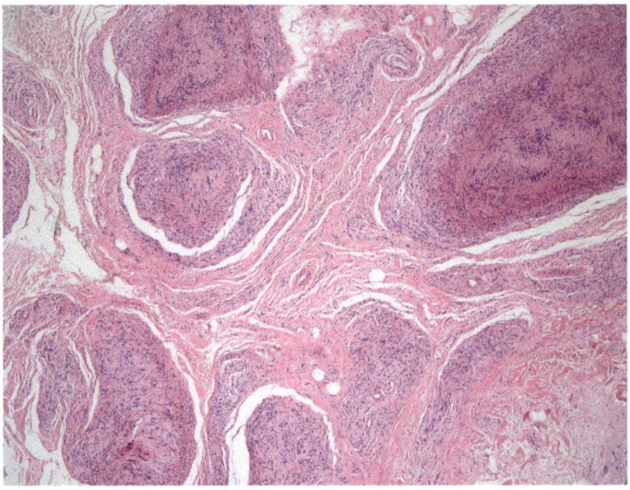

Fig. 4.66 Plexiform schwannoma: large nodules composed of Verocay bodies. The nodules are individually otherwise characteristic of schwannoma

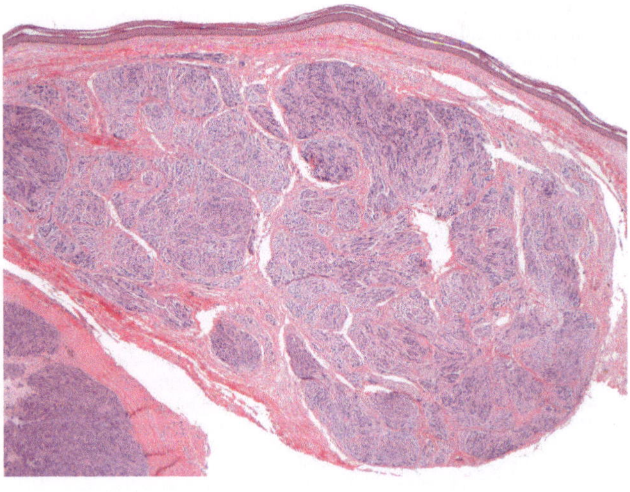

Fig. 4.67 Plexiform schwannoma: multiple nodules are separated by dermis and fibrous tissue. Some are surrounded by capsule

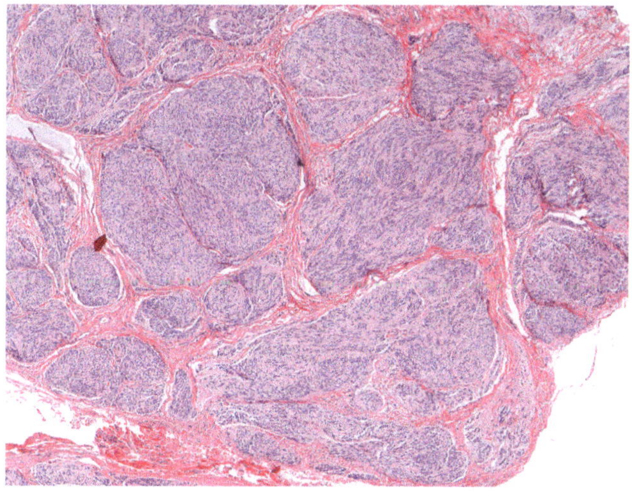

Fig. 4.68 Plexiform schwannoma: these variants, like cellular schwannoma, are often composed of Antoni A areas exclusively. Unlike the latter, plexiform schwannoma lacks the marked cellular density. Nuclear palisading is evident

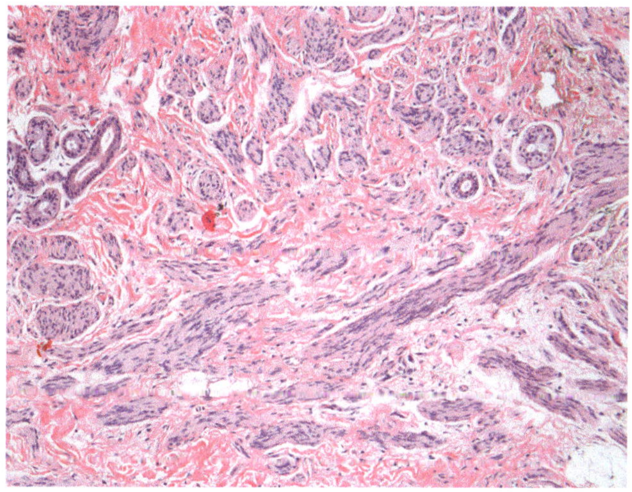

Fig. 4.69 Plexiform cellular schwannoma, congenital type: a neoplasm from an infant composed of haphazardly arranged Schwann cell rich fascicles throughout the dermis. Unlike plexiform neurofibroma, there is no myxoid stroma. These neoplasms may be locally destructive and complete excision is warranted

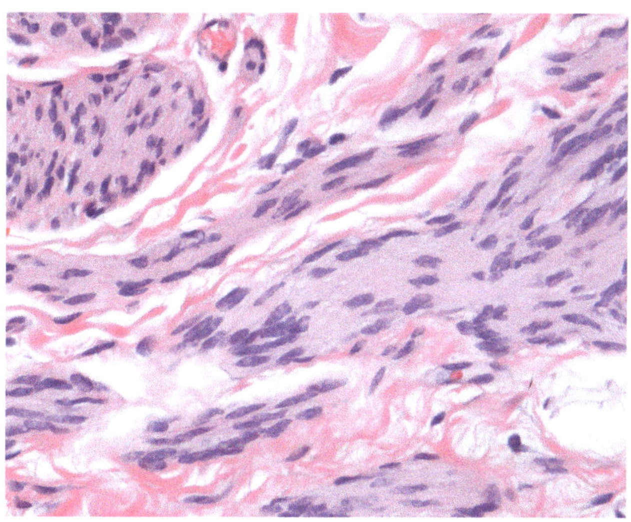

Fig. 4.70 Plexiform cellular schwannoma, congenital type: the Schwann cells are otherwise typical of schwannoma, with slender tapered nuclei and uniform fine chromatin

resembling normal nerve fibers (Figs. 4.69 and 4.70). The fascicles are haphazardly arranged and not encapsulated. At first glance they may resemble the bundles of smooth muscle hamartoma. Each fiber is composed exclusively of Schwann cells. The nuclei may be arranged at the periphery of each fascicle with a central zone of collagen-rich fibrillar cytoplasmic processes. Expanded fascicles may have large areas devoid of nuclei and resemble Verocay bodies. Mitotic figures may be present. Subcutaneous involvement may be evident. Normal nerve fascicles, presumably the "parent" nerve of origin may be identified at the deep aspect. The Schwann cells are positive for S-100 protein and type IV collagen (Fig. 4.71). Unlike other hamartomas, axons and perineurial cells are absent.

Pseudoglandular schwannoma is a rare morphologic variant of schwannoma, where the Schwann cells are arranged in tubular or gland-like structures (Figs. 4.72–4.74). These are true Schwann cells and not epithelial cells, demonstrated by immunohistochemical reactivity for S-100 protein, and negative staining for cytokeratins (Fig. 4.75). True glandular schwannoma as described represents a schwannoma with admixed epithelial glands. It is uncertain if this represents a form of bilineal differentiation or, more likely, entrapment of existing adnexal (eccrine or apocrine) glands.

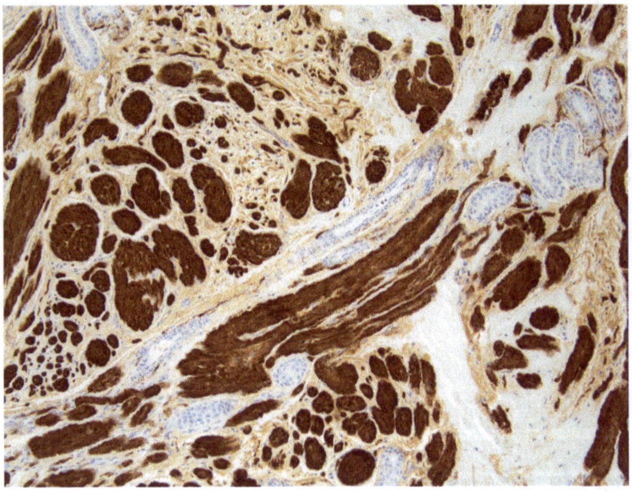

Fig. 4.71 S-100 protein in plexiform cellular schwannoma: the neoplastic cells of this and all variants of schwannoma show strong and diffuse nuclear and cytoplasmic staining. This differs from neurofibroma in which most (but not all) express this marker

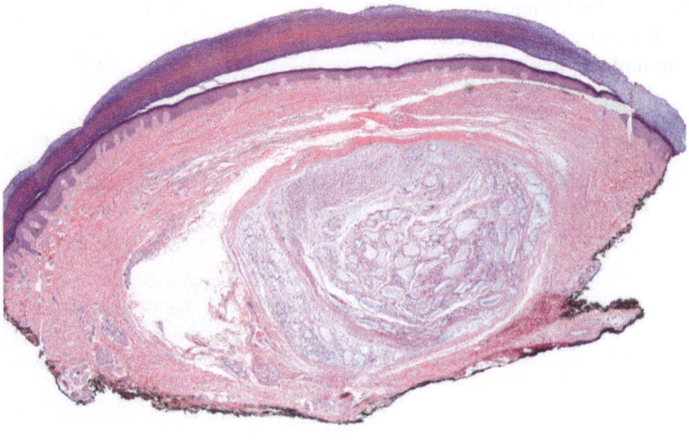

Fig. 4.72 Pseudoglandular schwannoma: a circumscribed dermal mass with a thick capsule and multiple ecstatic spaces resembling epithelial glands

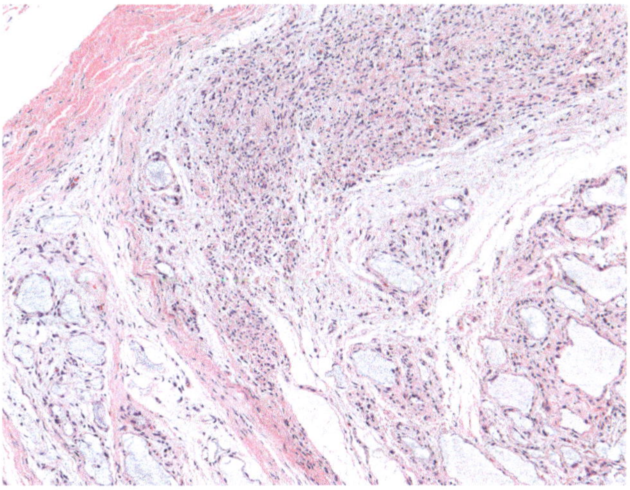

Fig. 4.73 Pseudoglandular schwannoma: granular basophilic material is present within the gland-like spaces. A diffuse spindle cells proliferation is present at the edge, resembling neurofibroma. The capsule and absence of axons is most characteristic of schwannoma however

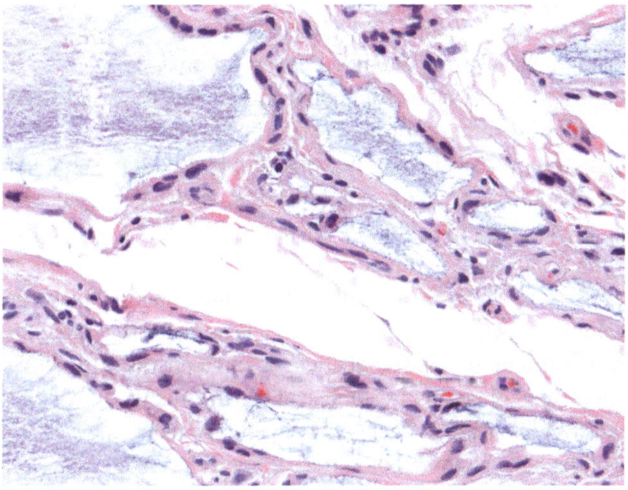

Fig. 4.74 Pseudoglandular schwannoma: the cystic structures are lined by epithelioid and spindled Schwann cells, which lack the orderly architecture of true epithelium

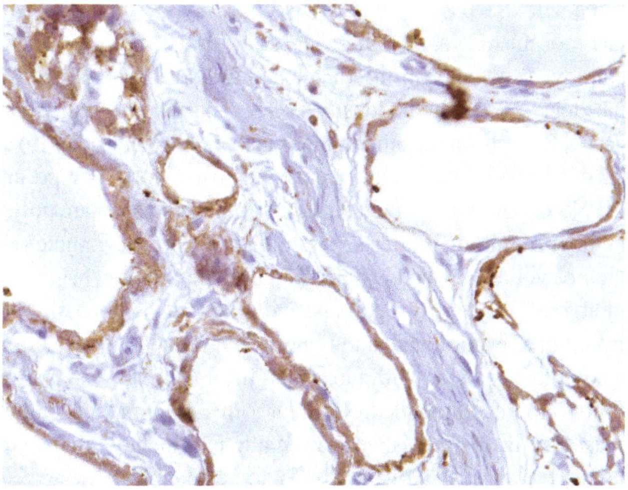

Fig. 4.75 Pseudoglandular schwannoma: S-100 protein expression by the lining Schwann cells confirms the nerve sheath lineage and absence of epithelium

Pigmented schwannoma is a descriptive term for a schwannoma composed of a population of cells containing melanin. *Psammomatous melanotic schwannoma* is a specific form with prominent psammoma bodies, associated with Carney complex. The Carney complex is an autosomal condition with risk of developing multiple lentigines, blue nevi, cutaneous and visceral myxomas, large cell calcifying Sertoli cell tumor of the testes, and pigmented nodular adrenal cortical hyperplasia.

Differential Diagnosis

The cardinal features that distinguish ordinary schwannoma from neurofibroma are discussed in the previous section. Plexiform variants are distinguished from plexiform neurofibroma by typical histologic and immunophenotypic features of ordinary solitary forms. Plexiform fibrohistiocytic tumor (PFHT) may be considered based on architecture at scanning magnification. However, at higher magnification PFHT is composed of epithelioid and multinucleated cells that lack expression of S-100 protein. The distinction of cellular schwannoma from MPNST is among the most difficult diagnostic challenges in cutaneous neural pathology, and established criteria distinguishing them are not yet well defined. In general, cellular schwannomas should have relatively uniform and monotonous nuclei and pleomorphism should raise concern for MPNST. Nevertheless, some MPNST have very little cytologic atypia or pleomorphism, and other criteria must be employed to establish the diagnosis. In addition, the degree of cellular density is very similar in each. Necrosis on the other hand is also more typical of MPNST. Marked mitotic activity also favors MPNST; however, as mentioned above, a precise number of mitotic figures separating these entities are not yet established. Therefore, a combination of atypia, cell density, necrosis, and mitotic activity should be employed, and if any doubt remains, a complete excision with clear margins and close follow-up recommended. Cellular schwannoma must also be distinguished from malignant melanoma; however, this distinction is somewhat less arduous as nonmelanotic schwannomas are negative for markers like HMB45 and Melan-A, and histologically encapsulated as opposed to melanomas.

Granular Cell Tumor

Definition, Classification, and Histogenesis

Granular cell tumor is a benign lesion with ultrastructural and immunohistochemical features of Schwann cell differentiation. The exact etiology of granular cell tumor remains debatable. Many authorities believe it represents a Schwann cell neoplasm with degenerative changes.

Clinical

Granular cell tumor may arise at any cutaneous site. Mucosa may also be affected. The tongue is one of the most frequently affected sites. Cutaneous forms are usually solitary; however, multiple forms may present in African-American individuals. Nodules may be verrucous or ulcerated. Rapid growth can be suggestive of a rare malignant granular cell tumor.

Histopathology

Most granular cell tumors are poorly delineated nonencapsulated proliferations of the dermis (Fig. 4.76). The lesional cells are arranged in cords and nests, which can have an infiltrative or plexiform growth pattern (Fig. 4.77). Intraneural or perineurial growth may be present. The cells are polygonal with small round, relatively uniform nuclei and small nucleoli (Fig. 4.78). The cells have abundant cytoplasm with conspicuous eosinophilic granules (Fig. 4.79). Some granules are large, globular, and surrounded by a clear space or halo. At first glance the cells may resemble smooth muscle, but are distinguished by their cytoplasmic features (Fig. 4.80). The granules, which are lysosomal bodies or phagosomes, are

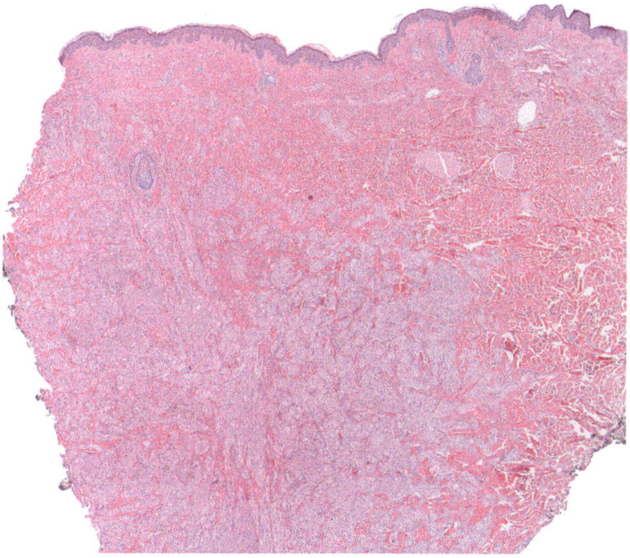

Fig. 4.76 Granular cell tumor: a rather diffuse proliferation of epithelioid cells arranged in small nests is present in the superficial deep dermis

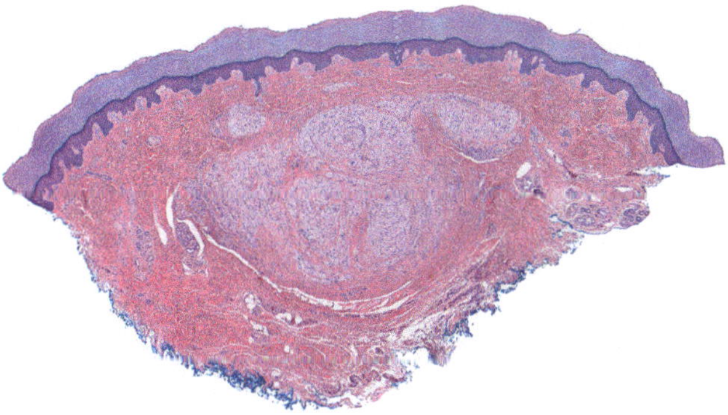

Fig. 4.77 Granular cell tumor: some variants have a plexiform or multinodular growth pattern

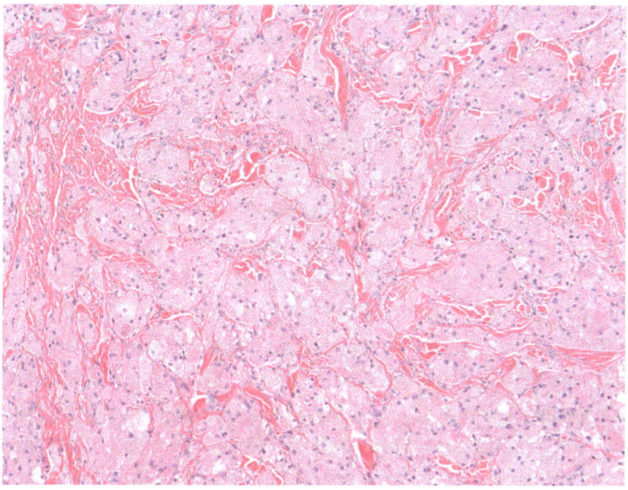

Fig. 4.78 Granular cell tumor: at medium magnification the nuclei have a monotonous appearance

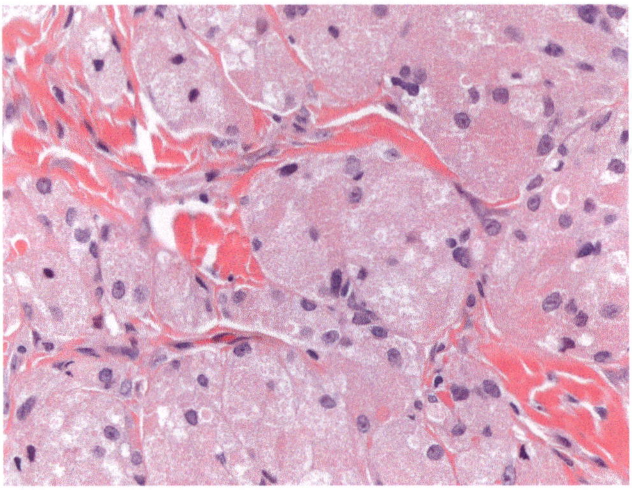

Fig. 4.79 Granular cell tumor: individual neoplastic cells are epithelioid with uniform round nuclei and small nucleoli that tend to orient at the periphery of the cells. There are innumerable small eosinophilic cytoplasmic granules. The latter corresponds to material with an ultrastructural appearance of myelin. Larger pink globules are also present

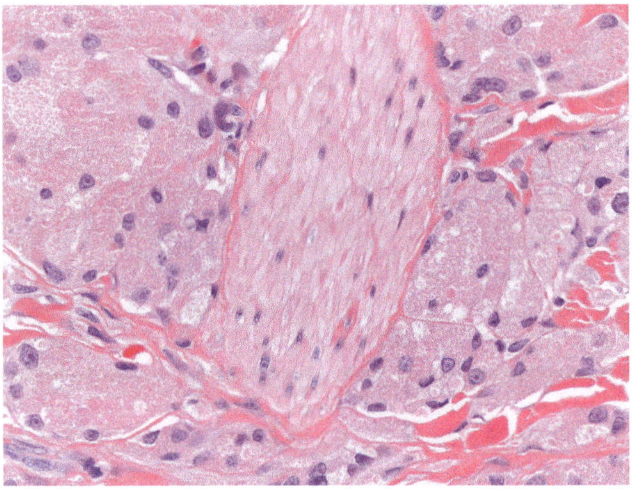

Fig. 4.80 Granular cell tumor adjacent to pilar smooth muscle: in contrast to the granular cell tumor, smooth muscle cells have glassy and pale eosinophilic cytoplasm with a syncytial appearance

PAS positive and diastase resistant. Ultrastructural features of myelin bodies may be detected. Mitotic figures are not uncommon and are not indicative of malignancy. Atypical mitotic figures however are unusual. Granular cell tumors are strongly and uniformly positive for S-100 protein (Fig. 4.81). The cells are also positive for vimentin, CD57, CD68, and microphthalmia transcription factor, but are negative for HMB45 and Melan-A. Of note, the overlying epidermis is often hyperplastic and rete ridges often have an irregular infiltrative appearance (Fig. 4.82). In some cases, the epidermis may mimic squamous cell carcinoma due to pronounced hyperplasia with mild nuclear atypia. This is often most prominent in the oral cavity. Hyperpigmentation of the basal keratinocytes may be observed, resembling lentigo or that observed overlying dermatofibroma.

Differential Diagnosis

Granular cell tumor must be distinguished from smooth muscle neoplasms such as leiomyoma. The latter is composed of spindle cells with cigar-shaped nuclei and eosinophilic cytoplasm with or without granularity. Smooth muscle cells are positive for smooth muscle actin and variably for desmin, and are negative for S-100 protein. Granular cell variants of fibrous histio-

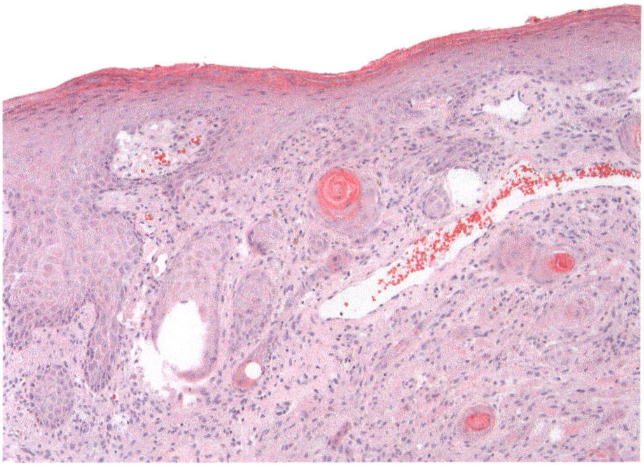

Fig. 4.81 Pseudoepitheliomatous hyperplasia: the epidermis is hyperplastic with extension of irregular projections of squamous cells into the dermis. This is a common finding overlying granular cell tumor. Lesions of the oral cavity in particular may be misdiagnosed as squamous cell carcinoma

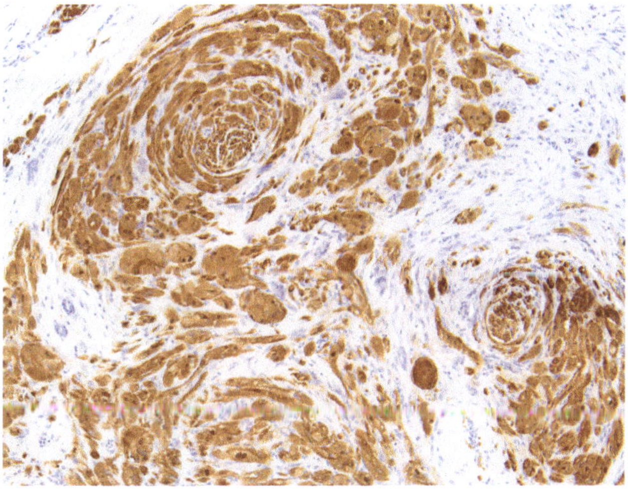

Fig. 4.82 S-100 protein is uniformly positive

cytoma/dermatofibroma are composed of spindle cells that do not form nests, and the lesional cells are negative for S-100 protein. Neurothekeoma may be composed of cells with granular cytoplasm, but are negative for S-100 protein.

Nerve Sheath Myxoma

Definition, Classification, and Histogenesis

NSM is a rare, benign neoplasm with ultrastructural and immunohistochemical evidence of Schwann cell lineage. In the past, NSM was classified as a variant of neurothekeoma; however, current recommendations state that the term NSM should only be used to define those neoplasms with evidence of Schwann cell differentiation in combination with the appropriate histologic changes. Neurothekeoma variants are discussed further in Chap. 6. One postulated histogenesis includes prominent mucin production within the endoneurium with eventual destruction of the normal Schwann cell–axon relationship (Fig. 4.83a, b for line drawings).

Clinical

NSM most often occurs on the distal extremities, most commonly the hands and fingers. There is no known gender or age predilection. Clinically, NSM appears as a nonspecific soft dermal papule or nodule. These may be flesh or pink colored,

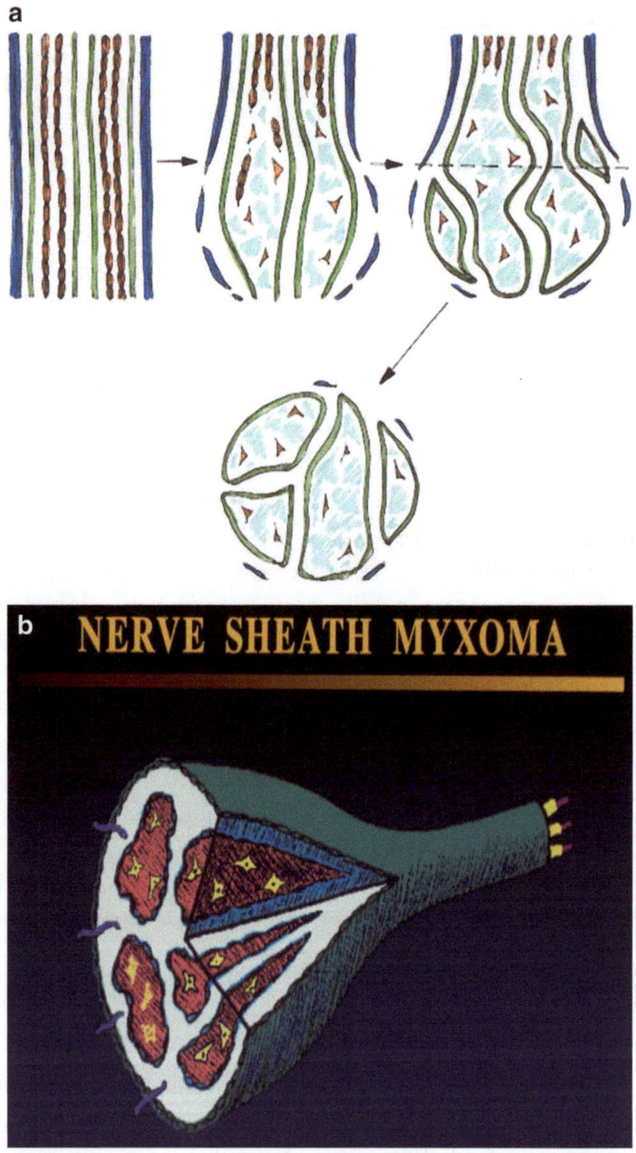

Fig. 4.83 (**a**, **b**) Schematic representation of *nerve sheath myxoma*. There is expansion of the fascicle by mucopolysaccharides, possibly derived from endoneurial stromal cells. The myxoid material displaces the normal nerve constituents. Schwann cells represent the neoplastic cells of nerve sheath myxoma, but are often present but in low numbers compared to the abundant stroma (artwork by ZA)

and are usually painless. Lesions may resemble nevi or dermatofibromas. There is no known association with a phakomatosis or endocrine disorders. Recurrence can occur following incomplete excision, but there are no known malignant counterparts.

Histopathology

At low magnification, NSM is composed of multiple well circumscribed highly myxoid expanded fascicles and/or nodules which are interconnected and sometimes encapsulated (Figs. 4.84 and 4.85). Each nodule contains variable numbers of spindled or epithelioid cells embedded in a markedly myxomatous stroma (Fig. 4.86). Spindle cells have bland ovoid nuclei and distinct eosinophilic cytoplasmic processes (Fig. 4.87). The cells may resemble histiocytes or have stellate dendritic processes (Fig. 4.88). Epithelioid cells have round nuclei with dense cytoplasm. The nuclei often have a degenerative appearance with irregular contours and vesicular chromatin. The

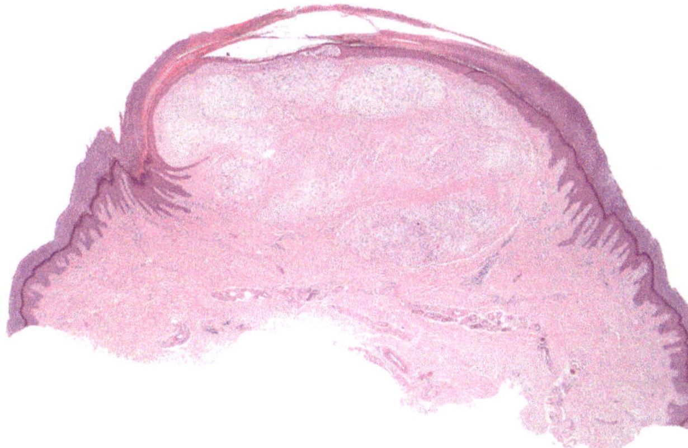

Fig. 4.84 Nerve sheath myxoma: a circumscribed multinodular dermal mass of acral skin. These most commonly arise on the hand. Schwann cells are arranged in discrete lobules that are separated by collagen

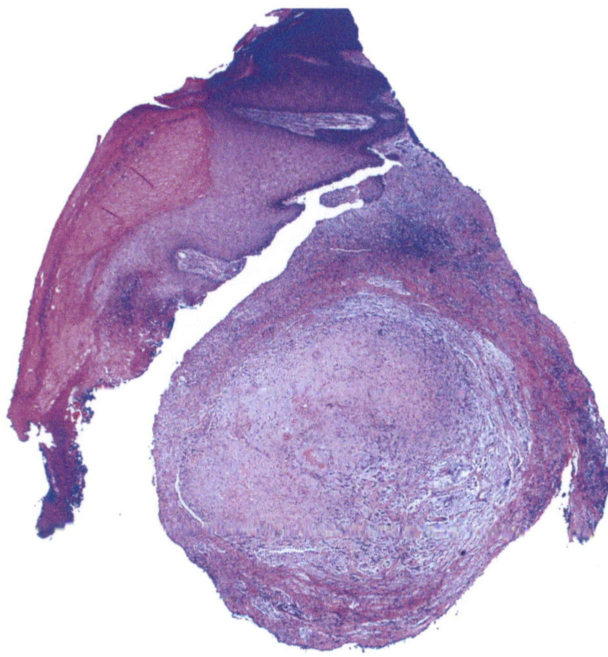

Fig. 4.85 Nerve sheath myxoma: an ulcerated acral mass that was recently biopsied is well circumscribed with an inflamed capsule

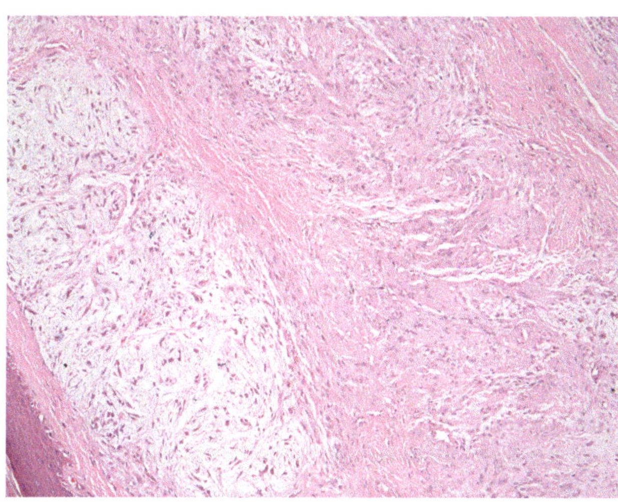

Fig. 4.86 Nerve sheath myxoma: the nodules have abundant myxoid stroma

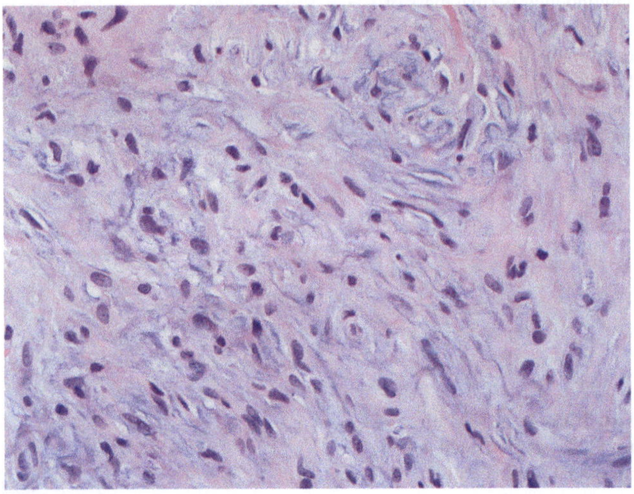

Fig. 4.87 Nerve sheath myxoma: many of the neoplastic cells are spindled. The nuclei are uniform with fine chromatin and mitotic figures are absent

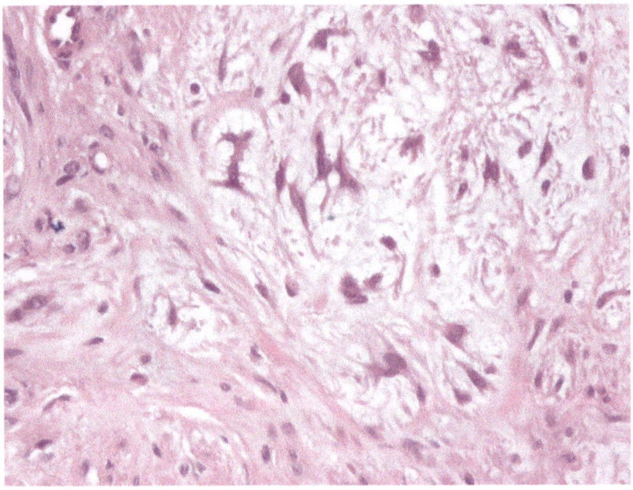

Fig. 4.88 Nerve sheath myxoma: The lesional cells may be dendritic, unlike the slender spindled Schwann cells of schwannoma and neurofibroma

cells may be arranged in cords, nests, or singly. Thin or delicate fascicles are sometimes present. Some cells may surround mucinous material in a pseudoglandular pattern, or appear to have cytoplasmic vacuoles (Figs. 4.89 and 4.90). Mitoses are absent or not conspicuous. Some tumors may be quite hypocellular, and the lesional cells may be difficult to visualize because of the abundant myxoid stroma. The neoplastic cells express S-100 protein and type IV collagen, typical of Schwann cells (Fig. 4.91), GFAP is also positive, but staining is usually fainter than the former antibodies (Fig. 4.92). Axons are not a component of this neoplasm. When encapsulation is preserved it is often highlighted by EMA stain.

Differential Diagnosis

NSM should be distinguished from myxoid variants of schwannoma and neurofibroma. The latter will have other features typically associated with these lesions. In particular, pseudoglandular schwannoma may resemble the ring-shaped cells surrounding myxoid material of NSM. Cells with the appearance of cytoplasmic vacuoles may raise consideration of soft tissue chordoma/parachordoma. The latter however is positive for cytokeratins and EMA, and negative for S-100 protein and GFAP. Extraskeletal myxoid chondrosarcoma is composed of thin cords and strands of epithelioid cells similar to NSM, but is

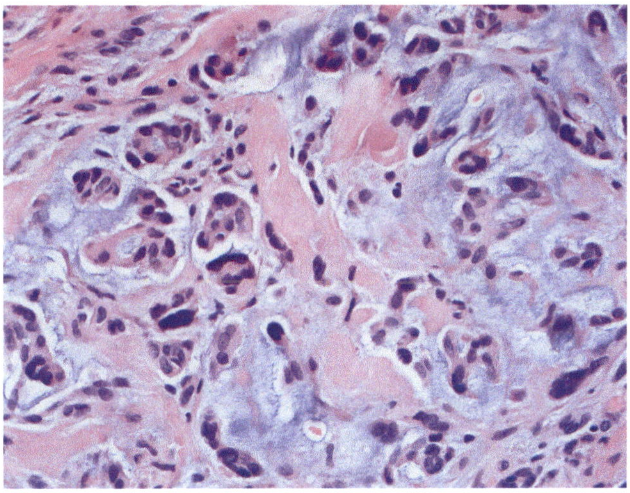

Fig. 4.89 Nerve sheath myxoma: epithelioid cells may be present. Some surround myxoid material, resembling pseudoglandular schwannoma

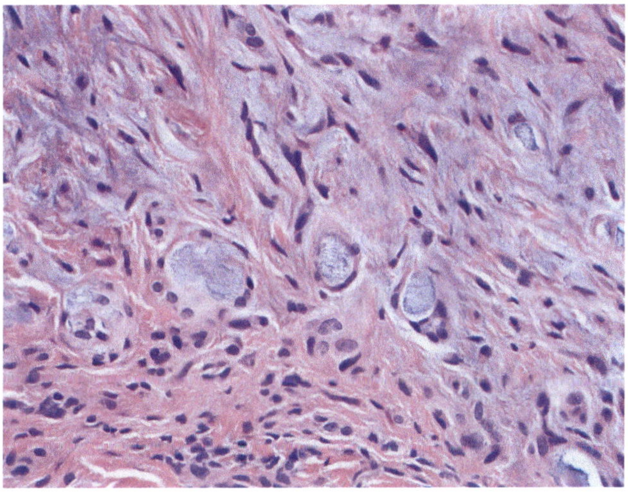

Fig. 4.90 Nerve sheath myxoma: cords of cells, some with entrapped myxoid material can mimic parachordoma. Absence of cytokeratins and EMA excludes the latter

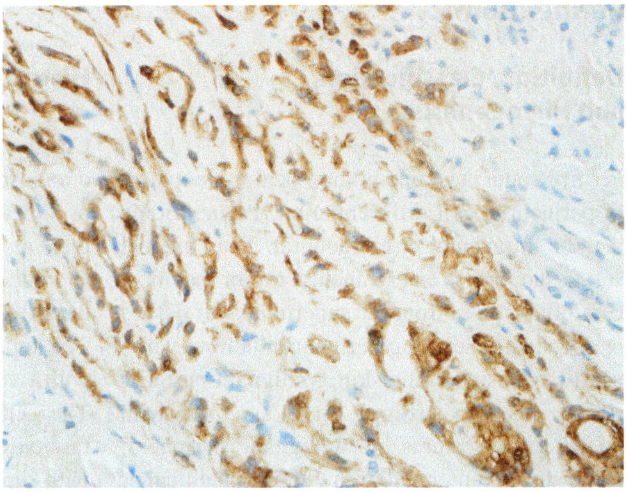

Fig. 4.91 Nerve sheath myxoma: the lesional cells are strongly positive for S-100 protein

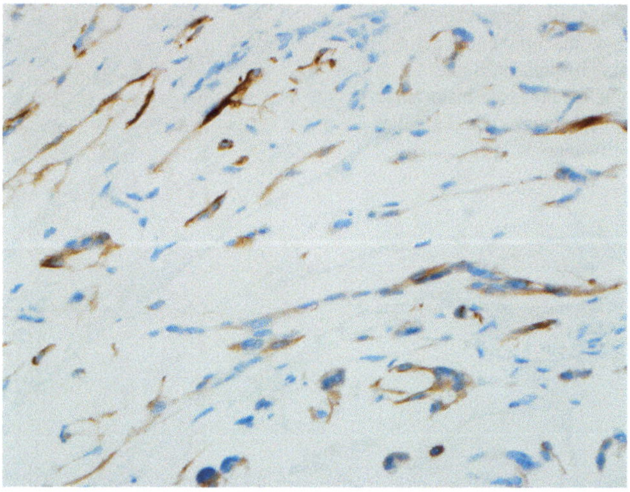

Fig. 4.92 Nerve sheath myxoma: the neoplastic cells also express GFAP although staining is often weaker than S-100

also negative for S-100 protein. NSM, particularly the hypocellular forms, can mimic nonneural lesions such as cutaneous mucinosis, ganglion cyst, and digital mucous cyst. These are negative for S-100 protein however. Angiomyxoma has abundant capillaries and is negative for S-100 protein. In addition, it lacks a multinodular growth pattern. Highly myxoid forms of neurothekeoma may be difficult to distinguish on H&E stained sections. Immunohistochemistry however can aid in this distinction, as neurothekeoma is negative for S-100 protein and GFAP. Often the lesional cells of neurothekeoma are plumper than the epithelioid cells of NSM.

Perineurioma

Definition, Classification, and Histogenesis

Perineurioma is an uncommon benign neoplasm of perineurial cell differentiation. Perineurioma may be intraneural or extraneural. The classical soft tissue form is an extraneural tumor that most commonly arises from the superficial soft tissues or subcutis. Sclerosing perineurioma however is nearly exclusive to the skin. Malignant perineurioma is an exceedingly rare sarcoma with microscopic features of malignant peripheral nerve sheath tumor and immunohistochemical or ultrastructural evidence of perineurial differentiation. To date no cases are reported in the skin.

Clinical

Classic perineurioma of the soft tissues shows a tendency for middle-aged patients, and usually arises on the extremities and trunk. Sclerosing perineurioma is commonly an asymptomatic slow-growing firm nodule on the hands of young adults. Males are more commonly affected. Intraneural forms (see below) are located in the deep soft tissues and the interested reader is referred to additional references given below. Perineurioma is benign with no significant rate of recurrence.

Histopathology

Classical soft tissue perineurioma consists of a circumscribed, but unencapsulated subcutaneous or soft tissue mass (Fig. 4.93). Dermal involvement alone can occur, but is not typical. The mass is composed of epithelioid and spindle cells with dense bipolar elongated cytoplasmic processes. The spindle cells characteristically form nodules with a whorled or storiform appearance (Fig. 4.94). The cells may also form intersecting or linear fascicles or have a lamellar growth pattern with clefs and cystic spaces (Figs. 4.95–4.97).

Fig. 4.93 Perineurioma: a soft tissue neoplasm with a thin collagenous capsule

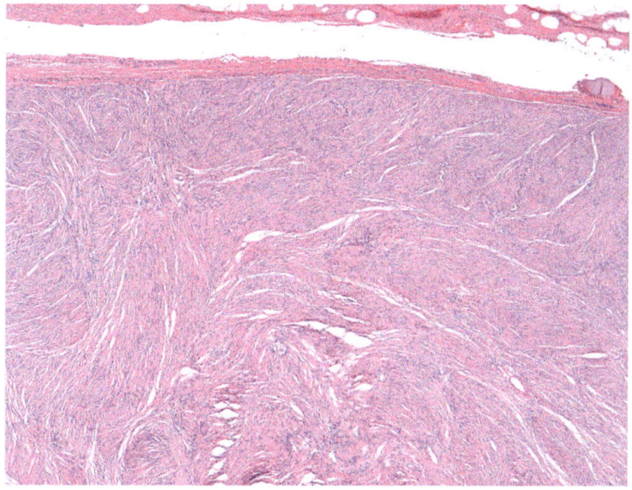

Fig. 4.94 Perineurioma: densely packed neoplastic perineurial cells arranged in lobules with a whorled and streaming appearance are separated by clefts

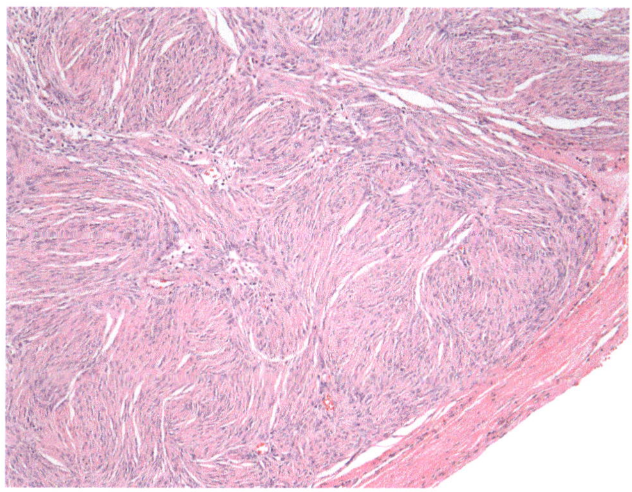

Fig. 4.95 Perineurioma: a microcystic appearance is common

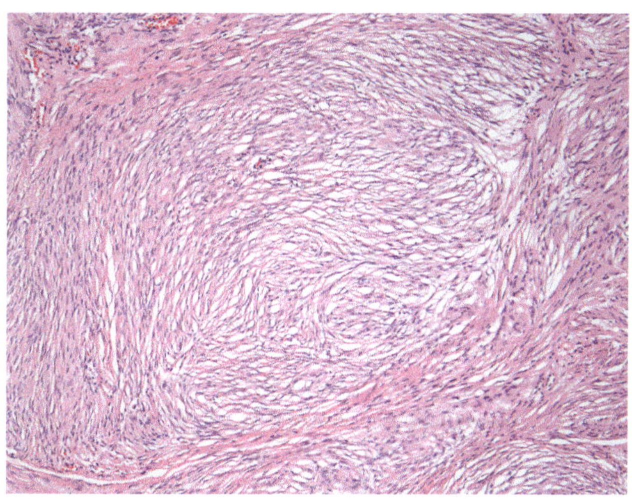

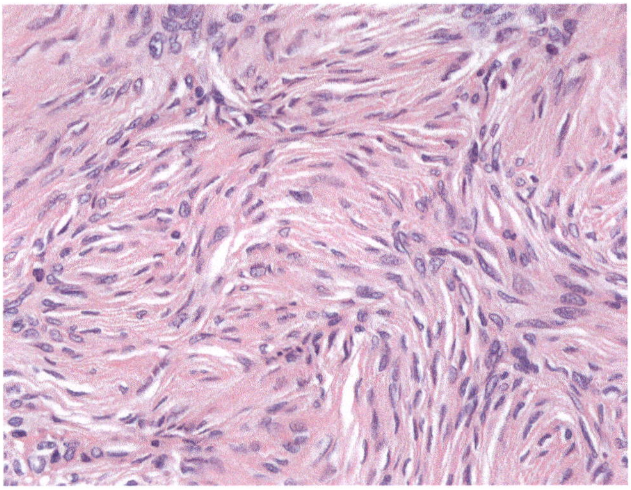

Fig. 4.96 Perineurioma: most cells have plump ovoid nuclei with fine chromatin, and dense eosinophilic bipolar cytoplasmic processes

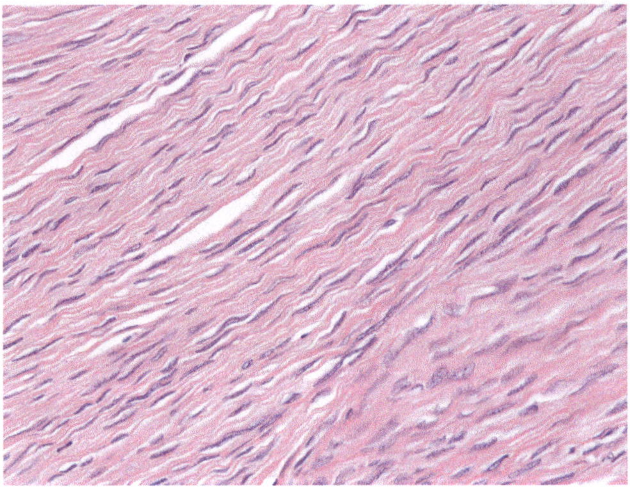

Fig. 4.97 Perineurioma: spindle cells arranged in parallel linear arrays mimics the arrangement of Schwann cells in normal nerve

The stroma may be myxoid, fibrous, or hyalinized. Mitotic figures are usually absent. Occasional lesions may be mitotically brisk but there is no documented increased risk of recurrence of malignant transformation. Some perineuriomas have more prominent epithelioid cytology with collagen-rich stroma (Figs. 4.98–4.102). Sclerosing perineurioma is an unencapsulated dermal or subcutaneous mass that may have a broad pushing border. It is composed of epithelioid cells arranged in cords, strands, or whorls, separated by a dense collagenous stroma (Fig. 4.103). Small blood vessels are usually prominent. The neoplasm involves the dermis, subcutis, or both. Reticular and intraneural variants are soft tissue lesions that do not commonly involve the skin. Reticular perineurioma consists of thin spindle cells separated by abundant myxoid stroma. Often the cells are arranged in a lattice-like network resembling small cysts. Intraneural variants, also known as localized hypertrophic neuropathy, present as an expanded swollen portion of nerve. Histologically, concentric layers of perineurial cells surround residual nerve fibers, likened to the appearance of an onion bulb.

By immunohistochemistry, perineurioma is positive for EMA, type IV collagen, GLUT-1, claudin-1, and laminin (Fig. 4.104). There may

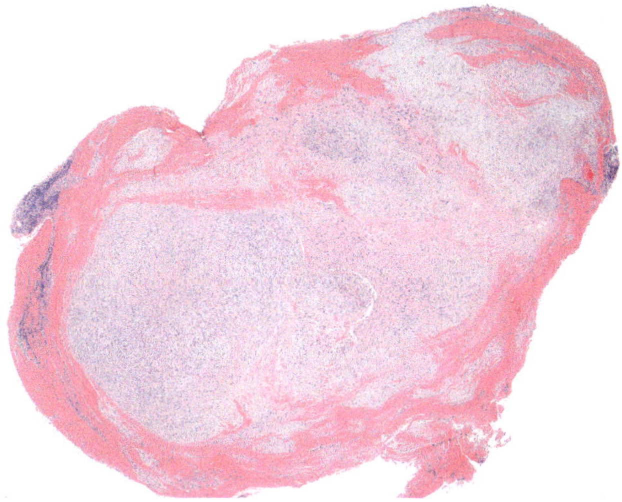

Fig. 4.98 Perineurioma: collagen-rich variants are common on acral skin and may involve the dermis, subcutis, or both

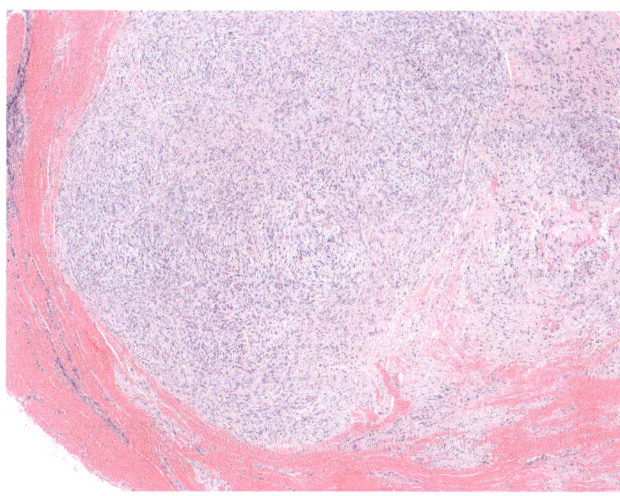

Fig. 4.99 Perineurioma: a thick collagenous capsule surrounds a nodule of spindle cells

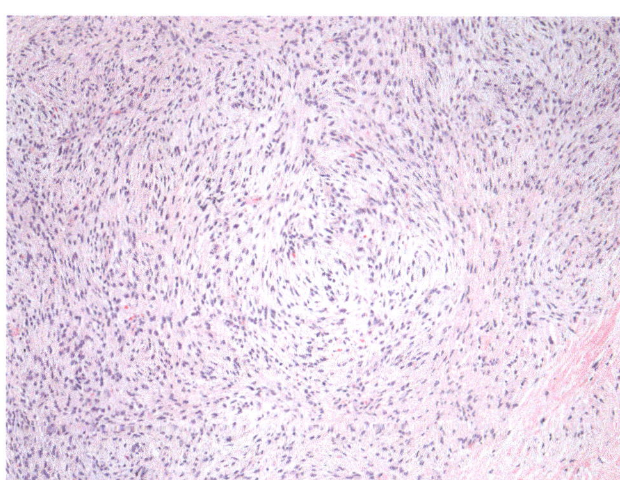

Fig. 4.100 Perineurioma: the spindle cells have thin elongated nuclei and are arranged in a whorled pattern

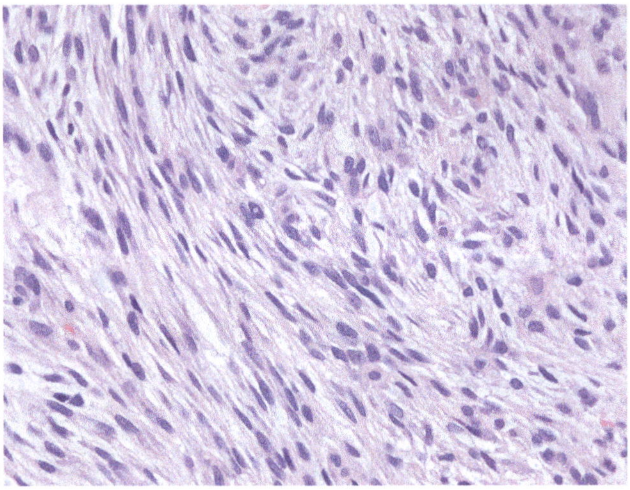

Fig. 4.101 Perineurioma: the neoplastic cells have uniform nuclei without atypia or mitotic activity

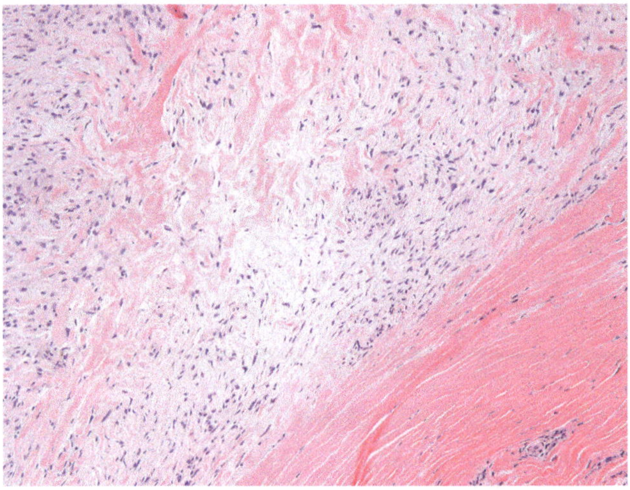

Fig. 4.102 Perineurioma: thick collagen fibers infiltrating between lesional cells

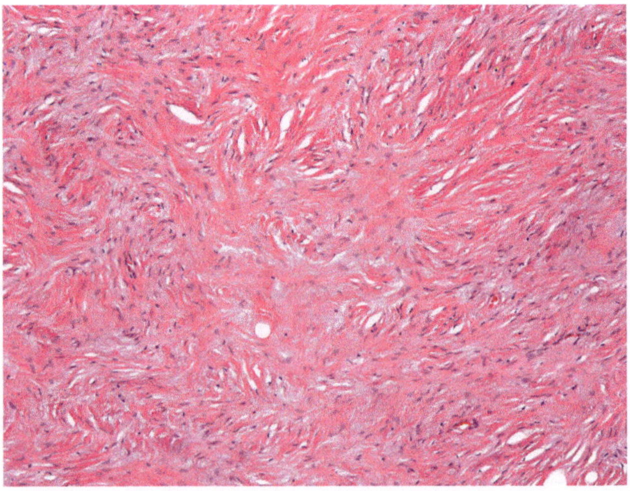

Fig. 4.103 Perineurioma: a sclerotic variant with abundant collagen and few lesional cells. Diagnosis of lesions with this morphology often requires immunohistochemistry for EMA, claudin, or GLUT-1

Fig. 4.104 Perineurioma: the cells of perineurioma are strongly positive for *EMA*, although in some cases expression is weak. The cells are negative for S-100 protein

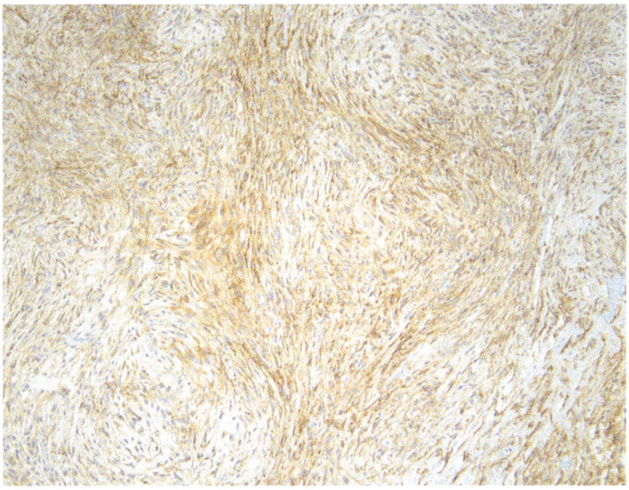

be focal or variable expression of pan-cytokeratin, CD34, and smooth muscle actin, the latter more common in sclerosing forms. S-100 protein, GFAP, and desmin are negative.

Differential Diagnosis

Classical soft tissue perineurioma is usually readily identified by its typical histopathologic and immunohistochemical characteristics. Expression of EMA distinguishes it from fibrohistiocytic proliferations including dermatofibroma and DFSP. Neurofibromas with lamellar architecture may resemble perineurioma. Expression of S-100 protein, variably distributed axons, and absence of diffuse EMA expression favors neurofibroma. There are however some lesions with combined morphologic and immunohistochemical features of neurofibroma and perineurioma, described as benign hybrid tumors, in which sharp distinction between the two is difficult. Sclerosing perineurioma should be distinguished from epithelioid variants of schwannoma and neurofibroma, sclerotic fibroma, and sclerotic or epithelioid forms of fibrous histiocytoma (dermatofibroma). Schwannoma and neurofibroma are S-100 protein positive. Sclerotic fibroma is usually less cellular, and those cells present are spindled and lack the corded arrangement of perineurioma. The lesional cells express CD34 and factor XIIIa and are EMA negative.

Lipoblastic Nerve Sheath Tumors

Lipoblastic nerve sheath tumor is a recently proposed descriptive term for an otherwise benign peripheral nerve sheath tumor with admixed adipocytes including lipoblast-like cells. The latter may resemble signet-ring cells of poorly differentiated adenocarcinoma. In the seminal description by Plaza et al., four of five cases involved the deep soft tissues and one presented in the subcutis. The underlying peripheral nerve sheath tumor shows features of schwannoma or neurofibroma. These likely represent morphologic variants of other peripheral nerve sheath lesions, akin to lipomatous NF.

Additional Reading

Neurofibroma

Fetsch JF, Michal M, Miettinen M. Pigmented (melanotic) neurofibroma: a clinicopathologic and immunohistochemical analysis of 19 lesions from 17 patients. Am J Surg Pathol. 2000;24:331.

Jokinen CH, Argenyi ZB. Atypical neurofibroma of the skin and subcutaneous tissue: clinicopathologic analysis of 11 cases. J Cutan Pathol. 2010;37:35.
Lin BT, Weiss LM, Medeiros LJ. Neurofibroma and cellular neurofibroma with atypia: a report of 14 tumors. Am J Surg Pathol. 1997;21:1443.

Schwannoma

Argenyi ZB, Goodenberg ME, Strauss JS. Congenital neural hamartoma ("fascicular schwannoma"). A light-microscopic, immunohistochemical and ultrastructural study. Am J Dermatopathol. 1990;12:283.
Berg JC, Scheithauer BW, Spinner RJ, Allen CM, Koutlas IG. Plexiform schwannoma: a clinicopathologic overview with emphasis on the head and neck region. Hum Pathol. 2008;39:633.
Laskin WB, Fetsch JF, Lasota J, Miettinen M. Benign epithelioid peripheral nerve sheath tumors of the soft tissues: clinicopathologic spectrum of 33 cases. Am J Surg Pathol. 2005;29:39.
Lim HS, Jung J, Chung KY. Neurofibromatosis type 2 with multiple plexiform schwannomas. Int J Dermatol. 2004;43:336.
Meis-Kindblom JM, Enzinger FM. Plexiform malignant peripheral nerve sheath tumor of infancy and childhood. Am J Surg Pathol. 1994;18:479.
Scheithauer BW, Woodruff JM, Erlandson RA. Tumors of the peripheral nervous system. In: Rosai J, Sobin LH, editors. Atlas of tumor pathology, series 3. Washington, DC: Armed Forces Institute of Pathology; 1999.
Woodruff JM, Scheithauer BW, Kurtkaya-Yapicier O, Raffel C, Amr SS, LaQuaglia MP, et al. Congenital and childhood plexiform (multinodular) cellular schwannoma: a troublesome mimic of malignant peripheral nerve sheath tumor. Am J Surg Pathol. 2003;27:1321.

Granular Cell Tumor

Vered M, Carpenter WM, Buchner A. Granular cell tumor of the oral cavity: updated immunohistochemical profile. J Oral Pathol Med. 2009;38:150–9.
Le BH, Boyer PJ, Lewis JE, Kapadia SB. Granular cell tumor: immunohistochemical assessment of inhibin-alpha, protein gene product 9.5, S100 protein, CD68, and Ki-67 proliferative index with clinical correlation. Arch Pathol Lab Med. 2004;128:771–5.
Kaiserling E, Ruck P, Xiao JC. Congenital epulis and granular cell tumor: a histologic and immunohistochemical study. Oral Surg Oral Med Oral Pathol Oral Radiol Endod. 1995;80:687–97.
Hatta J, Yanagihara M, Hasei M, Abe S, Tanabe H, Mochizuki T. Case of multiple cutaneous granular cell tumors. J Dermatol. 2009;36:504–7.

Nerve Sheath Myxoma

Fetsch JF, Laskin WB, Miettinen M. Nerve sheath myxoma: a clinicopathologic and immunohistochemical analysis of 57 morphologically distinctive, S-100 protein- and GFAP-positive, myxoid peripheral nerve sheath tumors with a predilection for the extremities and a high local recurrence rate. Am J Surg Pathol. 2005;29:1615.

Perineurioma

Emory TS, Scheithauer BW, Hirose T, Wood M, Onofrio BM, Jenkins RB. Intraneural perineurioma: a clonal neoplasm associated with abnormalities of chromosome 22. Am J Clin Pathol. 1995;103:696.
Fetsch JF, Miettinen M. Sclerosing perineurioma: a clinicopathologic study of 19 cases of a distinctive soft tissue lesion with a predilection for the fingers and palms of young adults. Am J Surg Pathol. 1997;21:1433.
Folpe AL, Billings SD, McKenney JK, Walsh SV, Nusrat A, Weiss SW. Expression of claudin-1, a recently described tight junction-associated protein, distinguishes soft tissue perineurioma from potential mimics. Am J Surg Pathol. 2002;26:1620.
Graadt van Roggen JF, McMenamin ME, Belchis DA, Nielsen GP, Rosenberg AE, Fletcher CDM. Reticular perineurioma: a distinctive variant of soft tissue perineurioma. Am J Surg Pathol. 2001;25:485.
Hornick JL, Fletcher CD. Soft tissue perineurioma: clinicopathologic analysis of 81 cases including those with atypical histologic features. Am J Surg Pathol. 2005;29:845.
Piña-Oviedo S, Ortiz-Hidalgo C. The normal and neoplastic perineurium: a review. Adv Anat Pathol. 2008;15:147.
Robson AM, Calonje E. Cutaneous perineurioma: a poorly recognized tumour often misdiagnosed as epithelioid histiocytoma. Histopathol. 2000;37:332.
Rosenberg AS, Langee CL, Stevens GL, Morgan MB. Malignant peripheral nerve sheath tumor with perineurial differentiation: "malignant perineurioma". J Cutan Pathol. 2002;29:362.
Yamaguchi U, Hasegawa T, Hirose T, Fugo K, Mitsuhashi T, Shimizu M, et al. Sclerosing perineurioma: a clinicopathological study of five cases and diagnostic utility of immunohistochemical staining for GLUT1. Virchows Arch. 2003;443:159.

Lipoblastic Nerve Sheath Tumors

Plaza JA, Wakely Jr PE, Suster S. Lipoblastic nerve sheath tumors: report of a distinctive variant of neural soft tissue neoplasm with adipocytic differentiation. Am J Surg Pathol. 2006;30:337.
Val-Bernal JF, González-Vela MC. Cutaneous lipomatous neurofibroma: characterization and frequency. J Cutan Pathol. 2005;32:274.

Malignant Cutaneous Neoplasms with Peripheral Nerve Differentiation

5

Keywords
Malignant peripheral nerve sheath tumors • Malignant schwannoma • Malignant granular cell tumor • Classification • Histogenesis • Diagnostic features • Differential diagnosis

Malignant Peripheral Nerve Sheath Tumor

Definition, Classification, and Histogenesis

Malignant peripheral nerve sheath tumor (MPNST) of the skin is a rare superficial sarcoma, capable of locally destructive growth and systemic metastasis. By definition, MPNST arises from a preexisting peripheral nerve sheath tumor or a nerve de novo. In the former circumstance, nearly all arise from a neurofibroma with a high association with the plexiform variant. Rare deeper variants of MPNST with epithelioid cytology may arise from schwannoma; however, this has not been well established in cutaneous forms. MPNST shows evidence of schwannian differentiation by immunohistochemical or ultrastructural methods. Rare forms with perineurial differentiation (malignant perineurioma) are described in soft tissues but so far not in the skin.

Clinical Findings

MPNST usually presents in adults. Examination reveals a firm nodule or tumor with or without epidermal alteration including erythema. These may be asymptomatic or associated with pain or paresthesias. Unlike other cutaneous sarcomas, MPNST is associated with metastasis, often to the lung and a guarded prognosis. MPNST commonly arises in patients with neurofibromatosis type 1. Cutaneous MPNST may be primary to the skin or represent secondary involvement from a deeper tumor.

Histopathology

At scanning magnification, MPNST appears as a hypercellular mass that may be circumscribed or diffuse (Figs. 5.1–5.8). Growth around nerves may be evident (Fig. 5.9). Neoplasms are composed of spindled and/or epithelioid cells. Spindle cells have irregular nuclei with coarse chromatin and usually inconspicuous nucleoli. The nuclei may be slender and wavy like those of schwannoma (Fig. 5.10), or plump and polygonal (Fig. 5.11). The degree of nuclear pleomorphism is variable. In some cases the spindle cells may be relatively monotonous, while in others there is marked variability in nuclear size and shape (Figs. 5.12–5.14). Usually the cells have very little cytoplasm, and thus nuclei of adjacent cells lie in close proximity to one another. The spindle cells are often arranged in long intersecting sweeping fascicles, which along with the

Z. Argenyi and C.H. Jokinen (eds.), *Cutaneous Neural Neoplasms*, Current Clinical Pathology,
DOI 10.1007/978-1-60327-582-8_5,

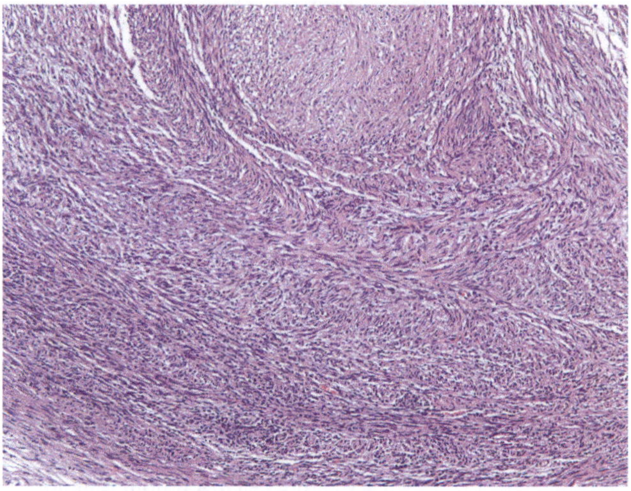

Fig. 5.1 Malignant peripheral nerve sheath tumor (MPNST): spindle cells arranged in dense sweeping fascicles with a herringbone appearance are typical

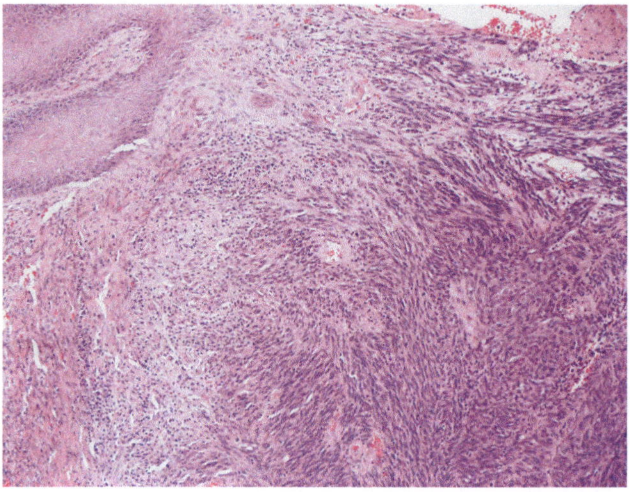

Fig. 5.2 MPNST: a dermal and subcutaneous variant extends to the epidermis. There are fascicles of hyperchromatic spindle cells

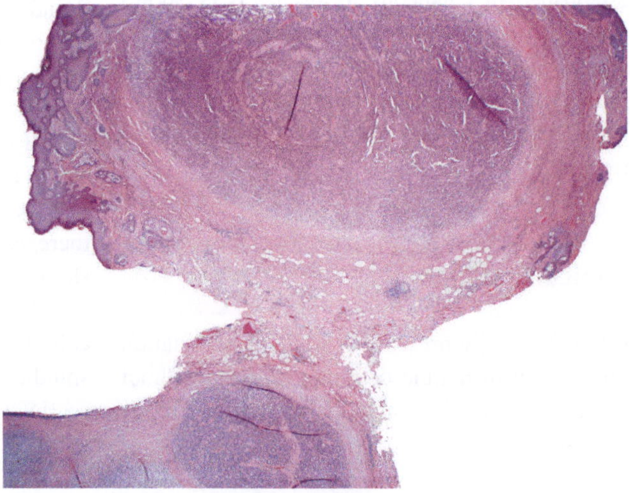

Fig. 5.3 MPNST: a polypoid dermal and subcutaneous mass from the face. The neoplasm consists of multiple circumscribed nodules

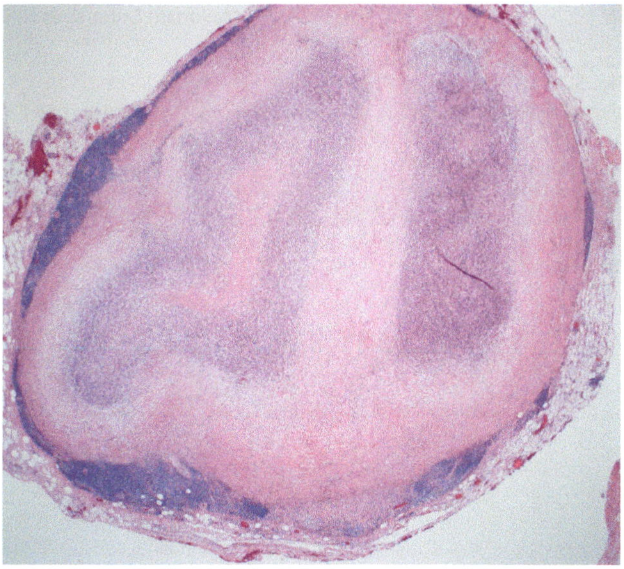

Fig. 5.4 MPNST: a well-circumscribed subcutaneous nodule that shows central geographic necrosis and is surrounded by lymphocytes at the periphery

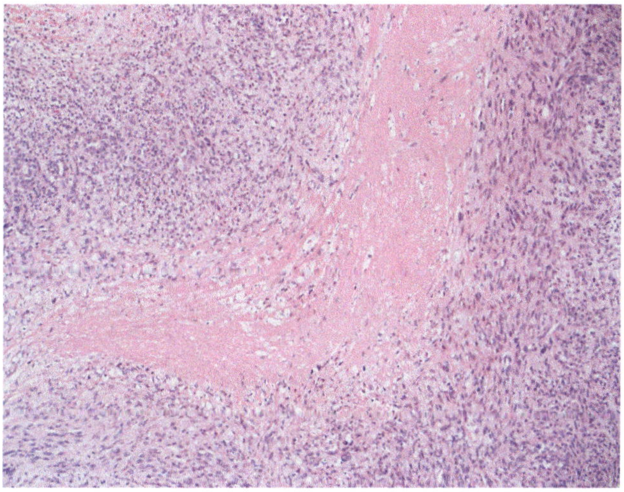

Fig. 5.5 MPNST: higher magnification of the necrotic areas with a rim of preserved malignant spindle cells

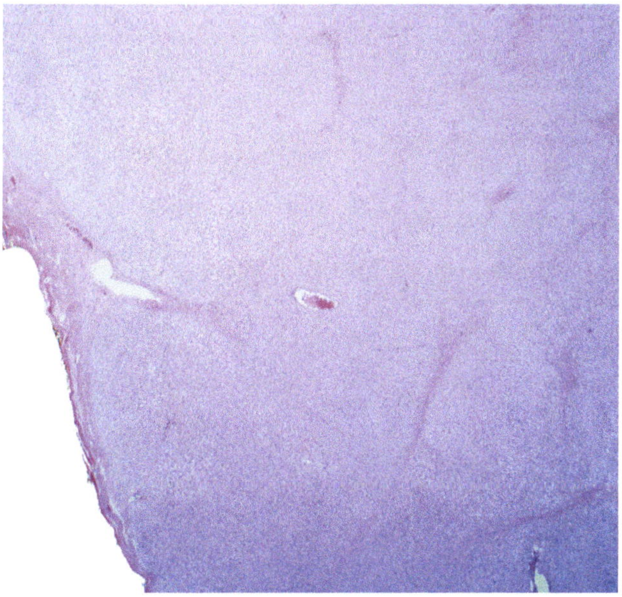

Fig. 5.6 MPNST: a subcutaneous neoplasm presenting as a well-circumscribed mass

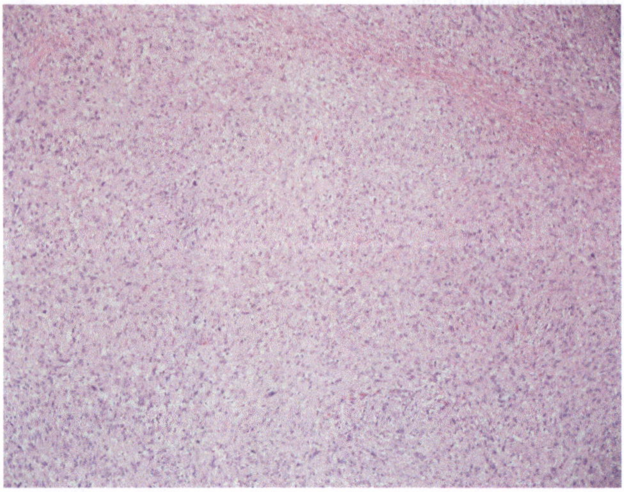

Fig. 5.7 MPNST: higher magnification shows an eosinophilic mass of polygonal cells and only moderate hypercellularity

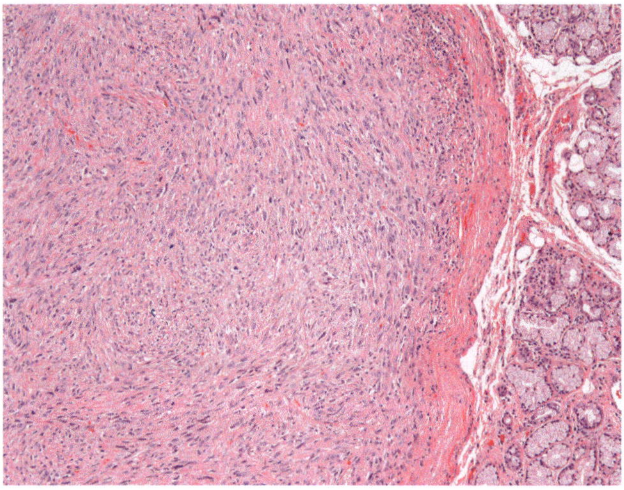

Fig. 5.8 MPNST: a well-circumscribed neoplasm of the lower lip adjacent to minor salivary gland. The neoplastic cells are arranged in vague fascicles

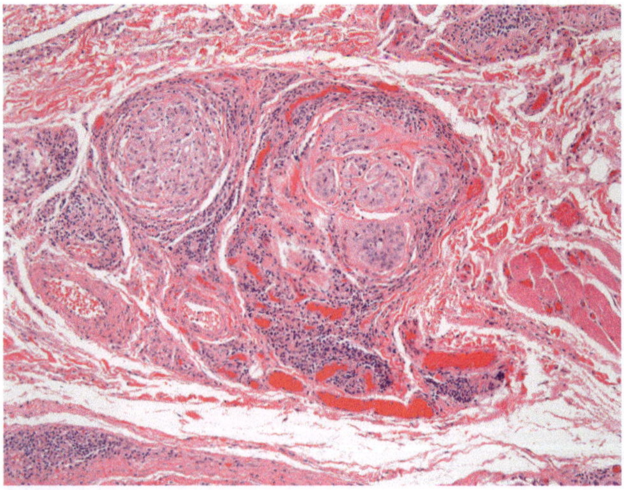

Fig. 5.9 MPNST: neoplastic cells are identified within adjacent nerve fascicles. In the absence of antecedent neurofibroma, intraneural growth of atypical polygonal cells in the absence of expression of melanocytic markers is highly suggestive of the diagnosis

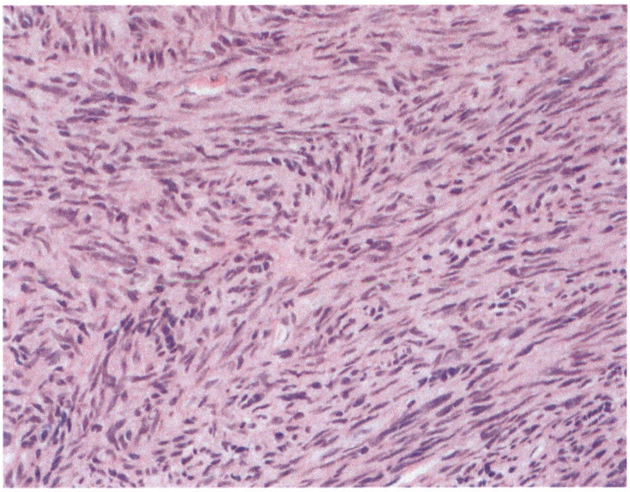

Fig. 5.10 MPNST: high magnification showing relatively homogenous spindle cells with elongated nuclei. Only rare mitotic figures were identified in this lesion

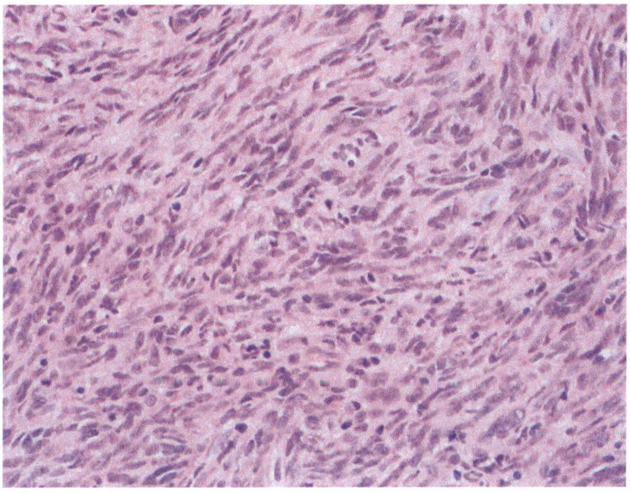

Fig. 5.11 MPNST: the cells have variable morphology. The same neoplasm as in Fig. 5.10 shows is composed of cells with more plump, ovoid nuclei

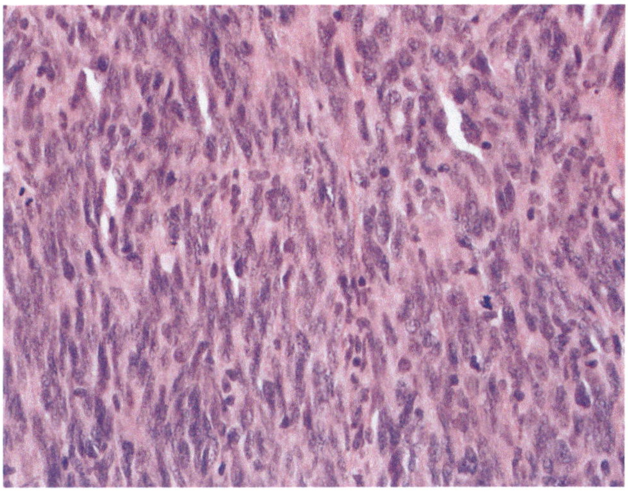

Fig. 5.12 MPNST: another example with marked hypercellularity. The nuclei are pleomorphic and have coarse chromatin with many mitoses

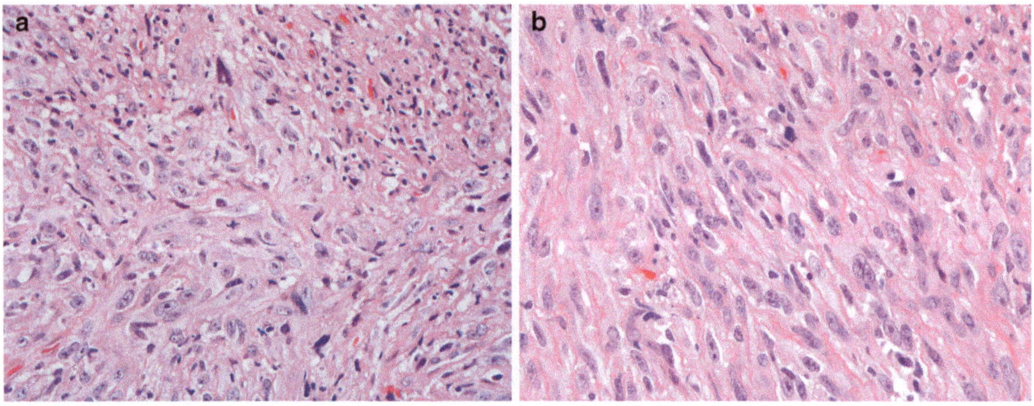

Fig. 5.13 (**a**, **b**) MPNST: in some lesions, the neoplastic cells are polygonal or epithelioid. The cells have irregular nuclei with large nucleoli. Variants with these cytologic features are often positive for S-100 protein. Absence of Melan-A or HMB45 distinguishes these from melanoma

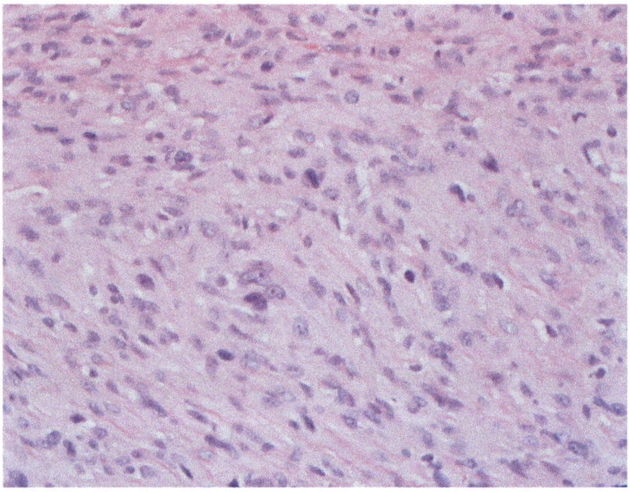

Fig. 5.14 MPNST: some tumors have only minimal pleomorphism with slightly irregular nuclei and abundant cytoplasm

variation of hyperchromasia of the nuclei suggest a herring-bone appearance resembling that of infantile fibrosarcoma. Mitotic activity is variable. In most circumstances, a brisk mitotic rate is encountered; however, in some forms, notably those with minimal atypia, mitoses may be difficult to find.

Epithelioid variants of MPNST are less common. On occasion, these may arise as a nodular proliferation within a neurofibroma (Figs. 5.15 and 5.16). In these, the malignant cells have round to polygonal hyperchromatic nuclei, sometimes with prominent nucleoli (Fig. 5.17a, b). Cytoplasm is scant. The cells lack cohesive properties but form a circumscribed nodule with associated necrosis or hyalinized stroma, distinct from the surrounding neurofibroma. Mitotic activity is often present, and often brisk. Rare variants contain adipocytic or lipoblast-like cells. Grading of primary superficial MPNST is currently not well characterized.

MPNST shows evidence of schwannian differentiation. However, expression of S-100 protein is variable and dependent on the morphologic subtype. Epithelioid variants of MPNST are commonly positive for S-100 protein. However, expression of this marker is only present in a subset of spindle cell MPNST, with some studies reporting reactivity in only 50–65% of cases. In fact, in the absence of epithelioid cytology, strong diffuse S-100 protein expression should raise consideration of malignant melanoma and

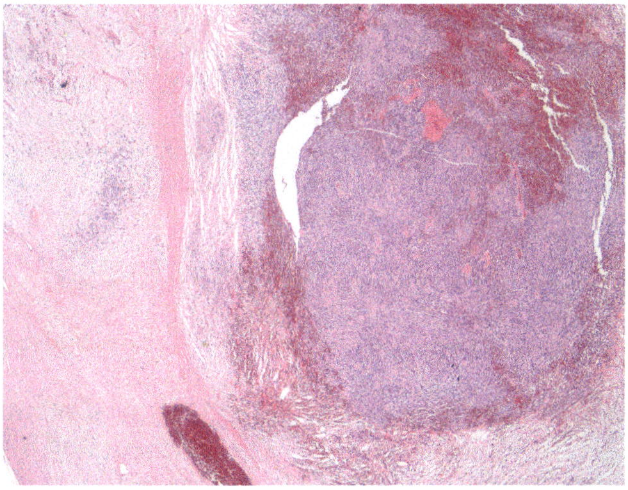

Fig. 5.15 MPNST arising in neurofibroma. The malignant cells form an expansile hypercellular nodule (*right*) separate from the neurofibroma (*left*) (higher magnification)

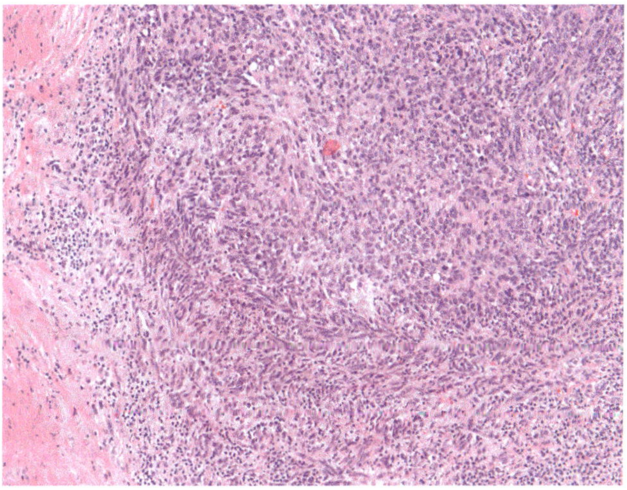

Fig. 5.16 MPNST arising in neurofibroma. The malignant cells form an expansile hypercellular nodule (*right*) separate from the neurofibroma (*left*) (higher magnification)

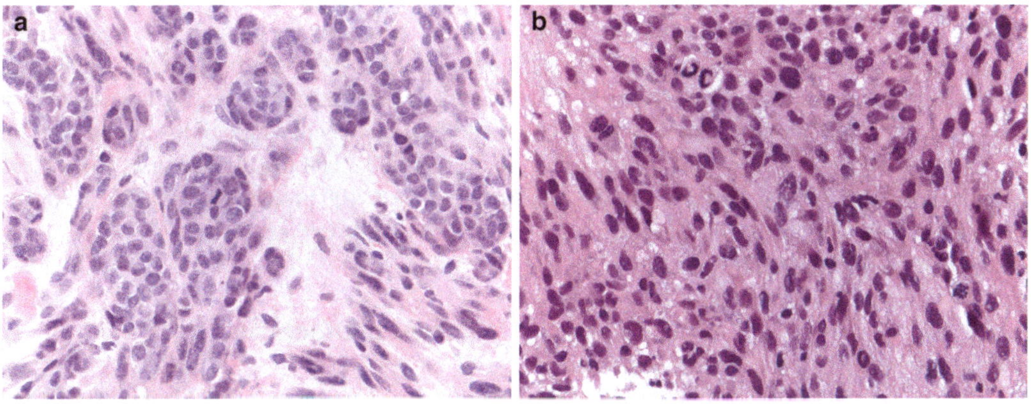

Fig. 5.17 (**a**, **b**) MPNST: the lesional cells have epithelioid features with hyperchromatic round nuclei and scant eosinophilic cytoplasm. Cytologically, they are nearly identical to those of malignant melanoma. Mitotic figures are present

additional melanocytic markers such as Melan-A or HMB45 should be routinely utilized. Expression of type IV collagen, CD57, p75 nerve growth factor receptor, and neuron specific enolase are less sensitive and specific indicators of neural differentiation, but can aid in establishing a diagnosis in the correct clinical and histopathologic context.

Differential Diagnosis

MPNST must be distinguished from cellular schwannoma and cellular or atypical neurofibroma. The distinction from cellular schwannoma may be very difficult in early forms, when encapsulation is still preserved as discussed in Chap. 4. Generally speaking, a combination of cellularity, nuclear atypia, dense fascicular growth, mitotic activity, and necrosis will aid in the distinction from neurofibroma. Atypical NF is only partially composed of pleomorphic cells and retains an intermingling of small spindle Schwann cells. Although atypical neurofibroma may have fascicular growth, the lesional cells are usually separated by stroma and lack the dense clustered or herringbone appearance of MPNST. The exact mitotic count to distinguish these still has not been established; however, greater than 1–3 mitotic figures in a tumor combined with these other features is considered more typical of MPNST. Melanoma is diffusely positive for S-100 protein and usually positive for Melan-A, HMB45, tyrosinase, or microophthalmia transcription factor, and ultrastructurally the cells contain melanosomes of various stages. Both MPNST and melanoma can express type IV collagen, however. Epithelioid variants of MPNST express podoplanin (D2-40), while this marker is absent in melanoma. Only a subset of spindle cell MPNST expresses podoplanin, however, so negative staining cannot exclude melanoma. Synovial sarcoma (SS) must be excluded, although this scenario applies more to soft tissue tumors secondarily extending to the superficial tissues. SS expresses keratin focally, EMA, and is negative for S-100. In cases where keratin is only focal or negative, FISH for the t(x; 18) fusion product may be contributory. MPNSTs are generally negative for muscle markers allowing distinction from leiomyosarcoma. However, a subset of soft tissue MPNST shows rhabdomyoblastic differentiation ("Triton tumor"). MPNST usually lacks the cytologic uniformity and storiform or whorled growth pattern of dermatofibrosarcoma protuberans; however, both may express CD34.

Malignant Granular Cell Tumor

Definition, Classification, and Histogenesis

Malignant granular cell tumors are exceedingly rare. The vast majority of granular cell tumors are benign. As discussed in Chap. 4, granular cell tumor is likely a Schwann cell neoplasm.

Clinical

Malignant granular cell tumor is a rapidly growing tumor. Some obtain large size, and ulceration may be present.

Histopathology

Malignant granular cell tumor may have marked cytologic atypia, increased mitotic activity, including atypical forms, and necrosis. An infiltrative growth pattern may be observed, but this is also common in benign variants. In some malignant variants, however, the microscopic features are indistinguishable from the benign form. Knowledge of the clinical presentation may be the only indication of the malignant nature of the tumor. Like the benign granular cell tumor, malignant variants are positive for S-100 protein and vimentin. They are negative for HMB45 and Melan-A.

Differential Diagnosis

Granular cell tumor must be distinguished from smooth muscle neoplasms like leiomyoma and leiomyosarcoma.

Additional Reading

Malignant Peripheral Nerve Sheath Tumor

George E, Swanson PE, Wick MR. Malignant peripheral nerve sheath tumors of the skin. Am J Dermatopathol. 1989;11:213.

Thomas C, Somani N, Owen LG, Malone JC, Billings SD. Cutaneous malignant peripheral nerve sheath tumors. J Cutan Pathol. 2009;36:896.

Tomas D, Franjić DB, Mijić A, Kruslin B. Malignant peripheral nerve sheath tumor with numerous signet-ring and lipoblast-like cells. J Cutan Pathol. 2009; 36:77.

6 Cutaneous Proliferations with Putative Neural Differentiation

Keywords
Putative neural tumors • Definitions • Classifications • Histogenesis • Diagnostic features • Differential diagnosis • Neurothekeoma • Merkel cell carcinoma • Cutaneous neuroendocrine carcinoma • Neurofollicular hamartoma

Neurothekeoma

Definition, Classification, and Histogenesis

Neurothekeoma (NTK) is a neoplasm of uncertain lineage. Previous descriptions classified NTK as cellular (immature) and myxoid (mature; classical) types based on the degree of cellularity. Currently, however, it is suggested that some highly myxoid and the previously described transitional or mixed variants with evidence of schwannian differentiation are better classified as dermal nerve sheath myxoma (see Chap. 4). NTK as currently classified on the other hand shows no convincing evidence of peripheral nerve lineage, and comprises a spectrum of tumors with variable degrees of cellularity and myxoid change. While the precise histogenesis is uncertain, some authors suggest this tumor may be of smooth muscle or fibrohistiocytic lineage. In general NTK is a benign neoplasm. While atypical forms exist, a true malignant variant has not yet been established.

Clinical Findings

NTK is most commonly a firm pink or tan asymptomatic nodule on the head and neck, although any anatomic site may be affected. There is a female predominance and younger individuals of the second and third decades tend to be affected. Incompletely excised lesions may recur. Presentation with multiple lesions is exceedingly rare.

Histopathology

NTK is a dermal proliferation composed of epithelioid or spindle cells arranged in fascicles, multiple nodules, or large sheets (Figs. 6.1–6.6). The lesion may have a nodular, well-circumscribed appearance (Figs. 6.7 and 6.8), and may extend to the subcutis. The lesional cells have round-to-oval nuclei, small nucleoli, and abundant yet poorly delineated dense eosinophilic cytoplasm (Figs. 6.9 and 6.10). Occasional granular cell variants may mimic granular cell tumor (Fig. 6.11). The chromatin often is concentrated around the nuclear membrane, and there is a prominent nucleolus. Multinucleated cells are not infrequent. Spindle cells with plump or ovoid nuclei are also common, and typically manifest as nests or whorls. Fascicles are less often evident (Figs. 6.12 and 6.13). The cells are often associated with sclerosis or grow in an infiltrative pattern between hyalinized collagen bundles (Figs. 6.14 and 6.15). Within the nodules, there are variable amounts of mucopolysaccharide-rich stroma (Figs. 6.16–6.22). Myxoid or mucinous

Z. Argenyi and C.H. Jokinen (eds.), *Cutaneous Neural Neoplasms*, Current Clinical Pathology,
DOI 10.1007/978-1-60327-582-8_6,

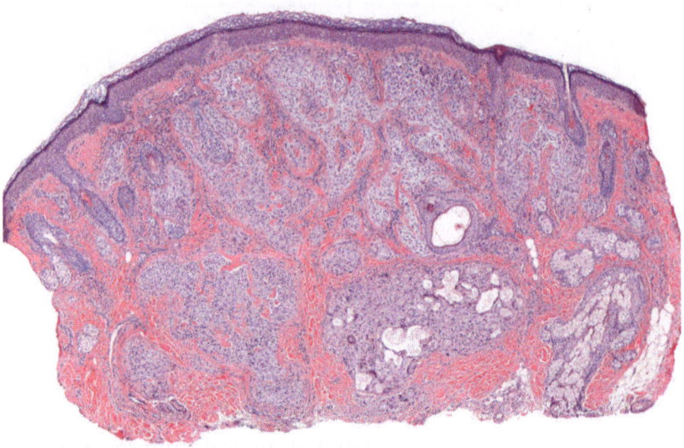

Fig. 6.1 Neurothekeoma (cellular): one of the common low-power appearances is that of nests and cords of epithelioid cells embedded in a sclerotic dermis

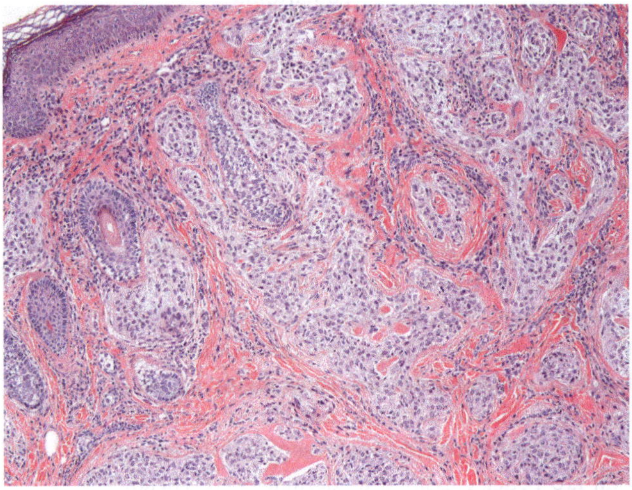

Fig. 6.2 Neurothekeoma (cellular): many cells are present in the nests and are separated by myxoid stroma

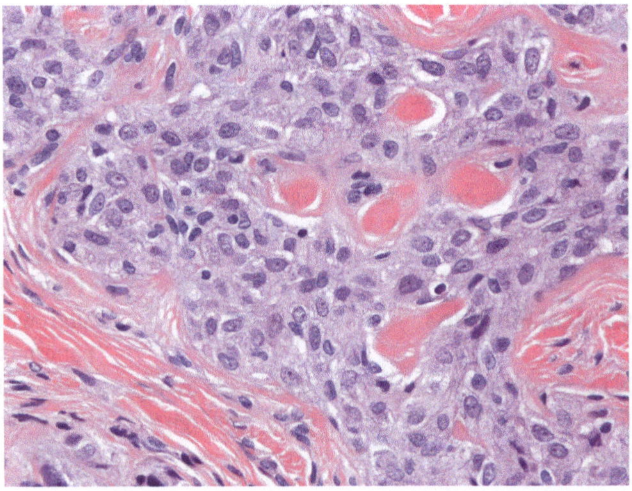

Fig. 6.3 Neurothekeoma (cellular): characteristic polygonal cells with round nuclei, fine chromatin, small nucleoli, and basophilic cytoplasm. Cell borders are indistinct. Mild variation in nuclear size and shape is common

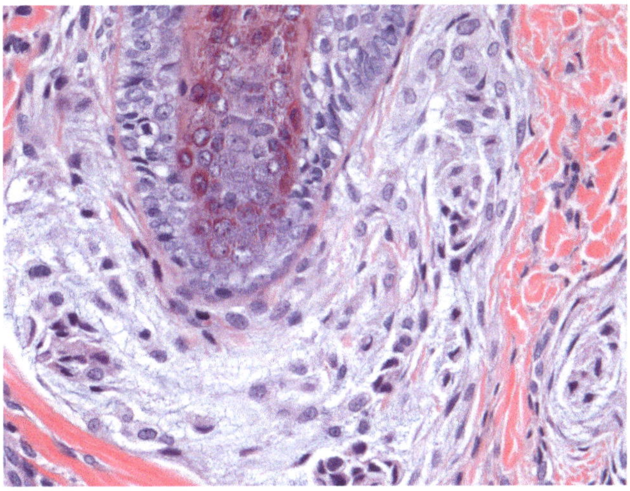

Fig. 6.4 Neurothekeoma (cellular): growth around hair follicles is common

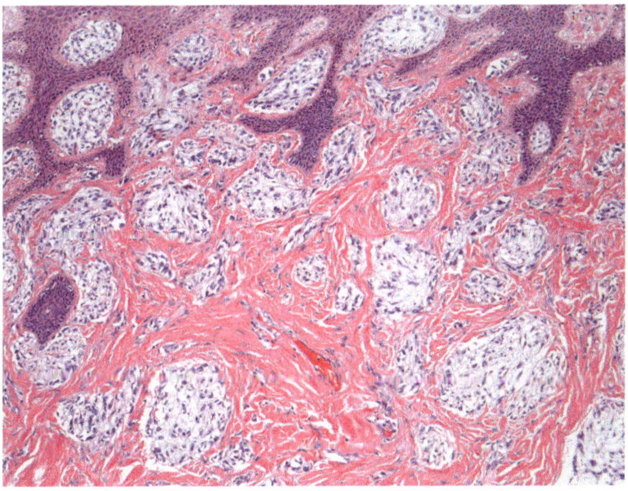

Fig. 6.5 Neurothekeoma (cellular): nodules of lesional cells in a sclerotic dermis. Myxoid stroma is more abundant in this example

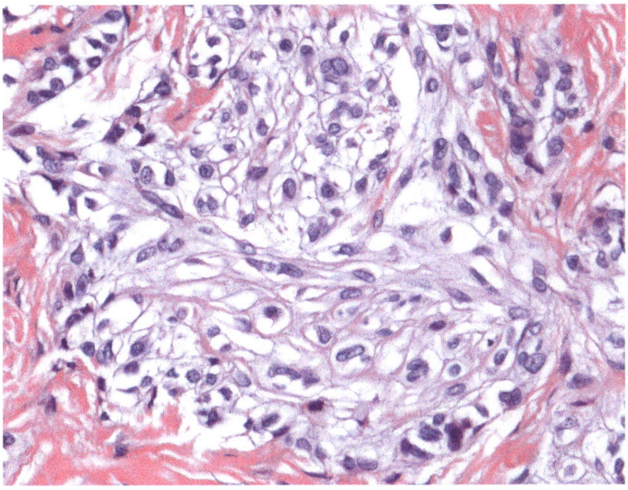

Fig. 6.6 Neurothekeoma (cellular): some cells have multilobular nuclei

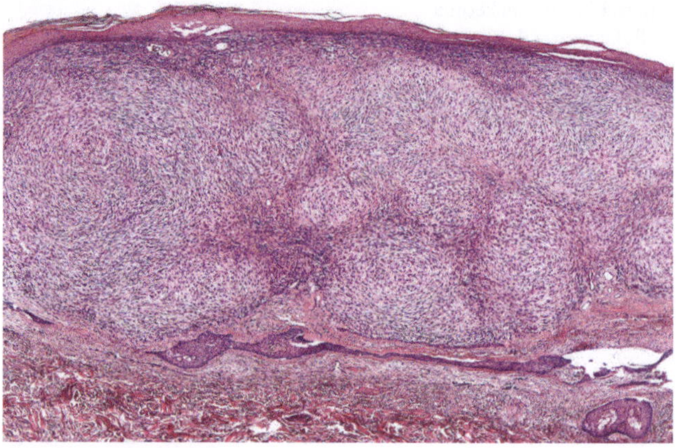

Fig. 6.7 Neurothekeoma (cellular): the nests can have a whorled appearance

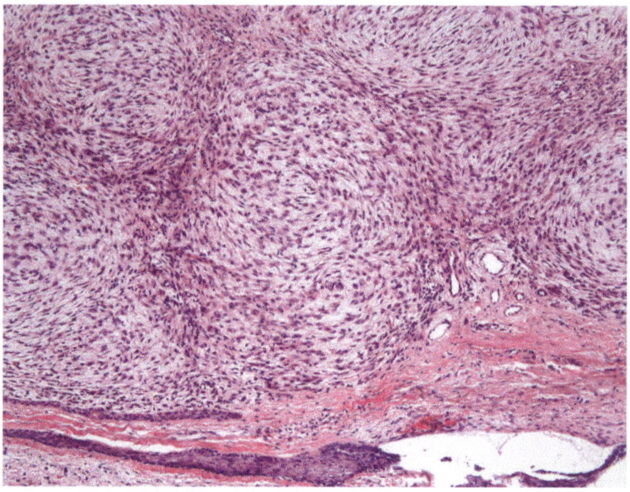

Fig. 6.8 Neurothekeoma (cellular): the neoplastic cells have a spindled appearance

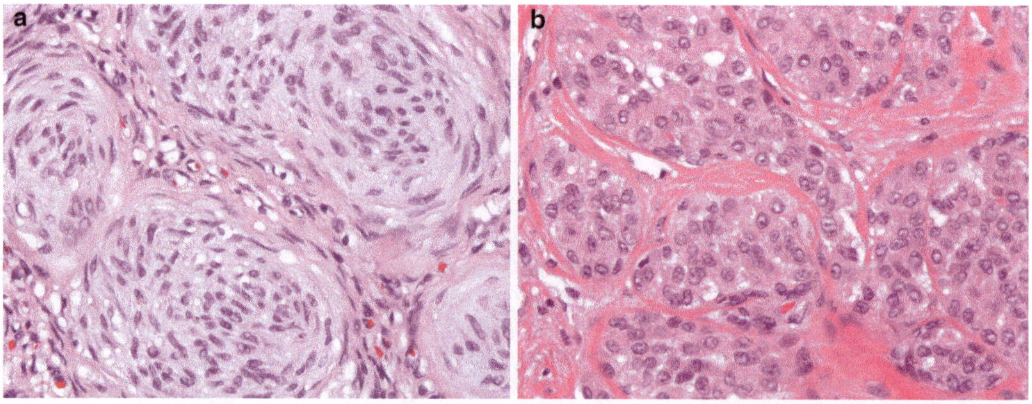

Fig. 6.9 (**a**, **b**) Neurothekeoma (cellular): epithelioid cells with pseudoinclusions arranged in small nests may mimic melanocytic nevus cells

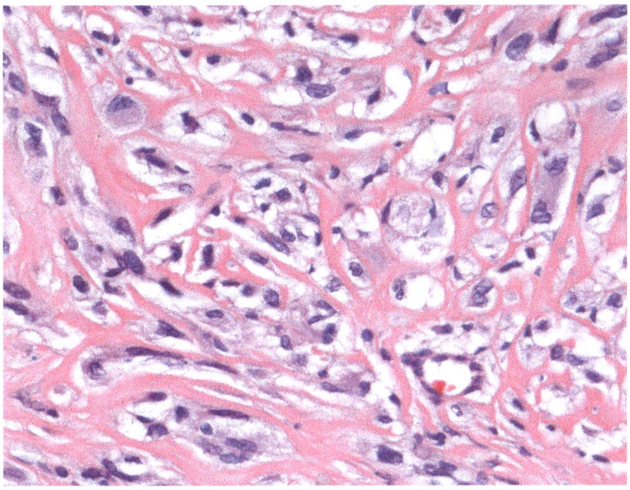

Fig. 6.10 Neurothekeoma: in some cases individual cells infiltrate between hyalinized collagens. Polygonal mononuclear and binucleate cells are typical

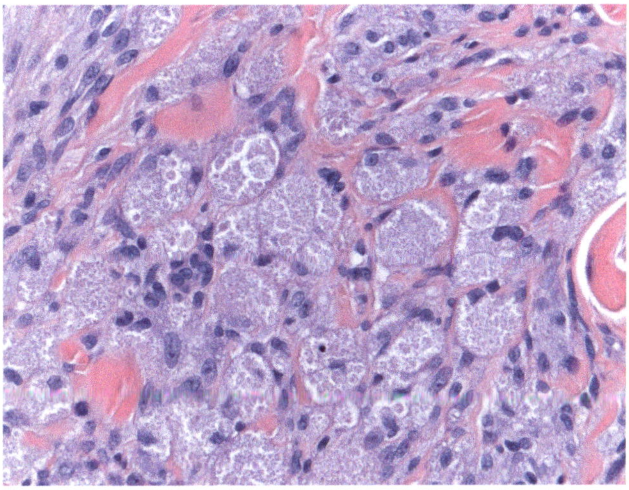

Fig. 6.11 Neurothekeoma: in this example the epithelioid cells have abundant granular cytoplasm. This is rare morphologic variant mimics granular cell tumor. Unlike granular cell tumor, neurothekeoma is negative for S-100 protein

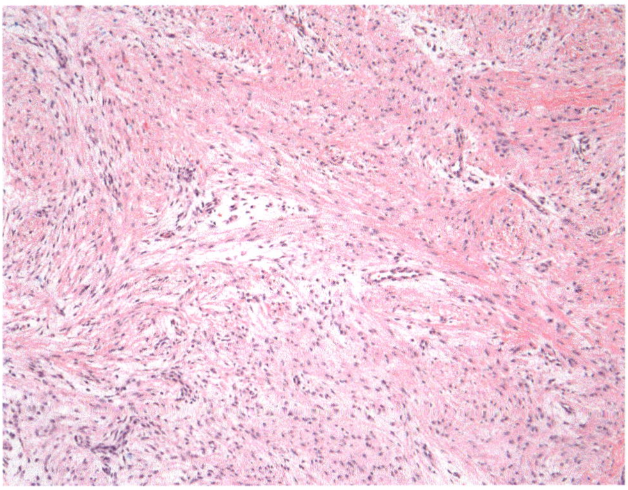

Fig. 6.12 Neurothekeoma: the so-called desmoplastic neurothekeoma consists of spindle cells with long eosinophilic cytoplasmic processes arranged in vague fascicles. These variants may resemble acral fibromyxoma

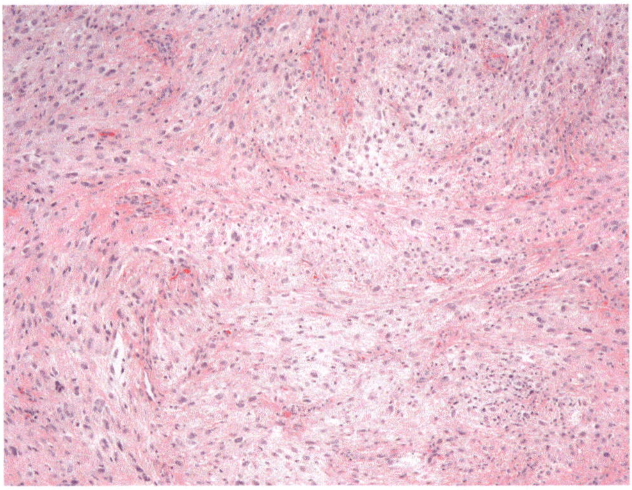

Fig. 6.13 Neurothekeoma: epithelioid or polygonal cells may also be arranged in nests with a broad sweeping appearance

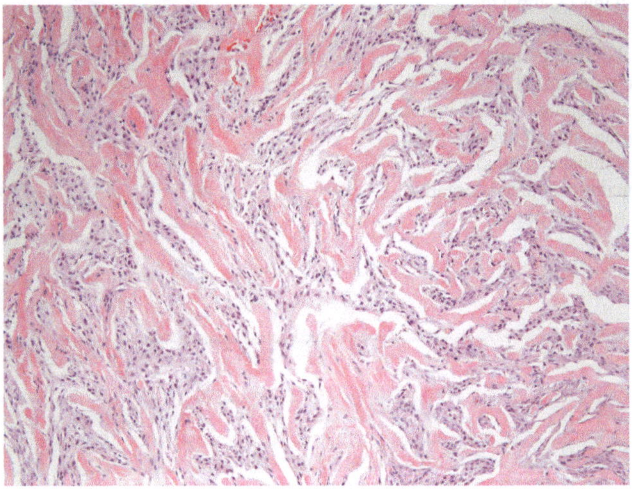

Fig. 6.14 Neurothekeoma: nests may have an infiltrative appearance separated by markedly hyalinized collagen

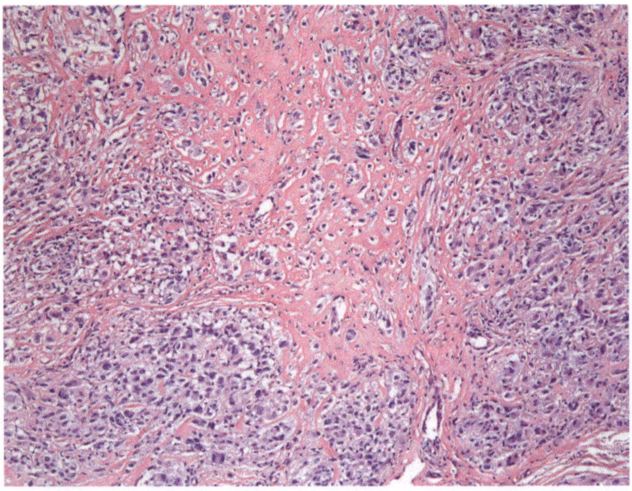

Fig. 6.15 Neurothekeoma: the stroma may be highly sclerotic

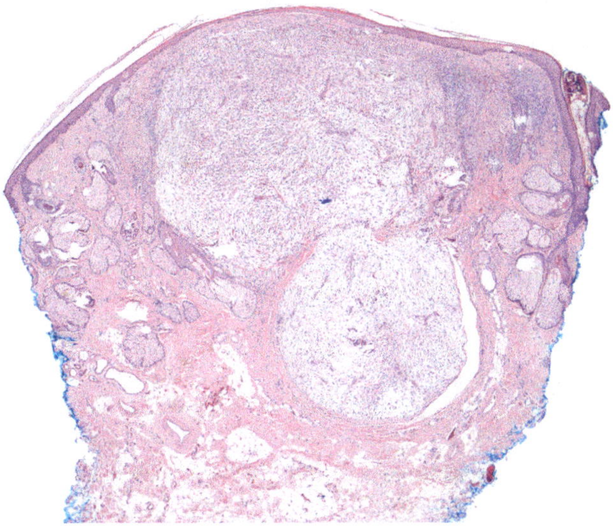

Fig. 6.16 Neurothekeoma (mixed cellular and myxoid): large nodules in the superficial and deep dermis with abundant myxoid stroma

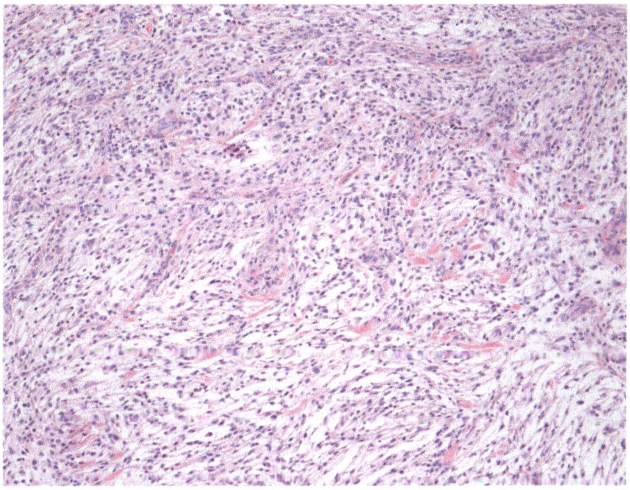

Fig. 6.17 Neurothekeoma (mixed cellular and myxoid): hypercellular areas (*top*) are present adjacent to myxoid hypocellular zones (*bottom*)

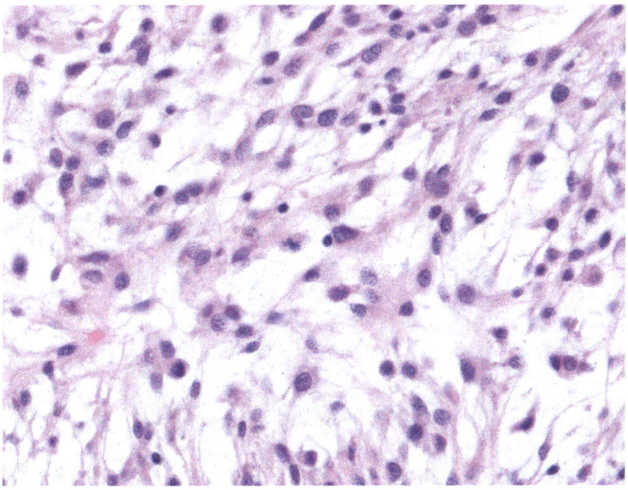

Fig. 6.18 Neurothekeoma (mixed cellular and myxoid): polygonal cells with dense eosinophilic cytoplasm in a myxoid stroma. Absence of S-100 protein expression distinguishes from nerve sheath myxoma

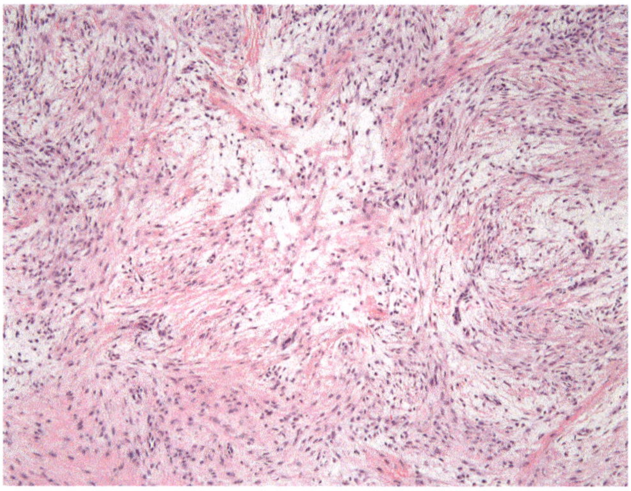

Fig. 6.19 Neurothekeoma (mixed cellular and myxoid): hypocellular areas with prominent myxoid change may resemble Antoni B areas of schwannoma

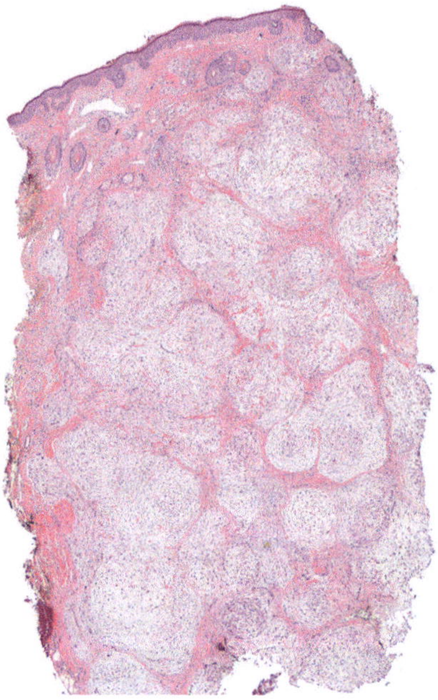

Fig. 6.20 Neurothekeoma (myxoid): closely opposed nodules rich in myxoid stroma occupy nearly the entire dermis

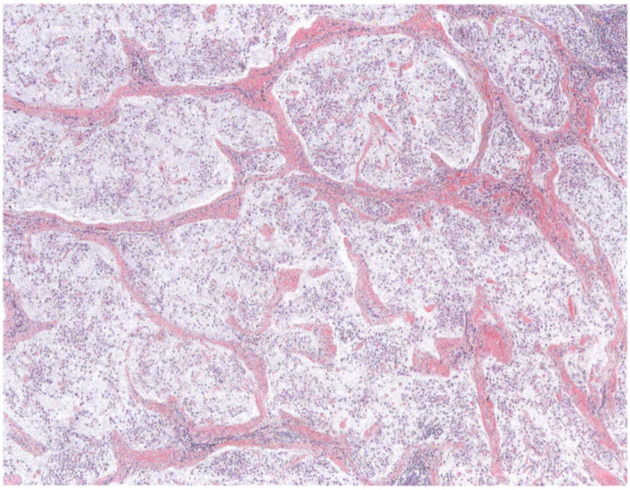

Fig. 6.21 Neurothekeoma (myxoid): nests of cells are divided by thick collagen fibers

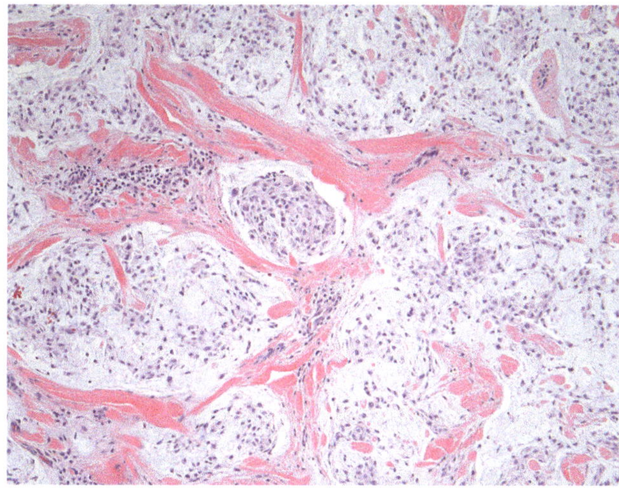

Fig. 6.22 Neurothekeoma (myxoid): most nodules contain abundant myxoid stroma. Invariably, however, hypercellular foci are present (*center*)

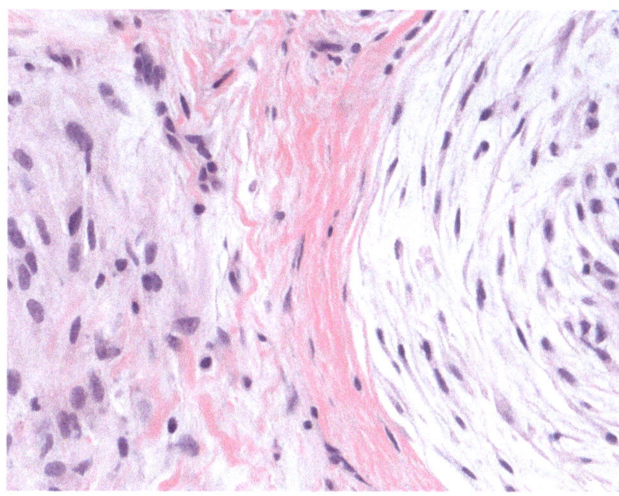

Fig. 6.23 Neurothekeoma (myxoid): epithelioid cells predominate in the hypercellular foci (*left*), whereas the highly myxoid nests often contain slender spindle cells (*right*)

material can be abundant with the nests, and the cells may have a floating appearance. The amount of ground substance is variable, and may be abundant, mimicking NSM, relatively sparse, or anywhere in between (Figs. 6.23 and 6.24). Occasionally, the overlying epidermis shows mild to moderate melanocytic hyperplasia or basal keratinocyte pigmentation. Mitotic figures can be conspicuous, ranging up to 15 per 10 high power fields in one study, and there may be variable cytologic atypia. These features do not appear predictive of recurrence or malignant potential. Although increased tumor size, nuclear pleomorphism, and mitotic activity may generate concern, these features do not appear predictive of recurrence. There is a variable and inconsistent immunohistochemical reaction pattern. NKI/C3, PGP 9.5, S-100A6 protein, and microophthalmia transcription factor are most commonly positive (Figs. 6.25 and 6.26). Many tumors express epithelial membrane antigen, neuron-specific enolase, CD68, and smooth muscle actin. S-100 protein, CD57 (Leu-7), and collagen type IV are absent.

Differential Diagnosis

Highly myxoid variants of NTK share overlapping features of dermal nerve sheath myxoma,

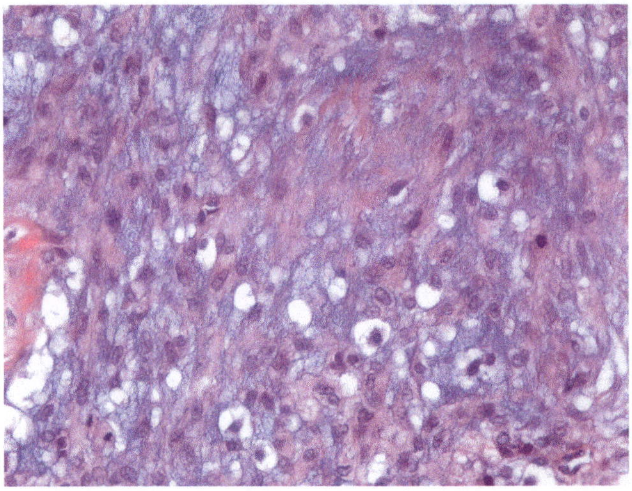

Fig. 6.24 Neurothekeoma (myxoid): abundant granular basophilic mucin. Rare mitotic figures are present (*right center*)

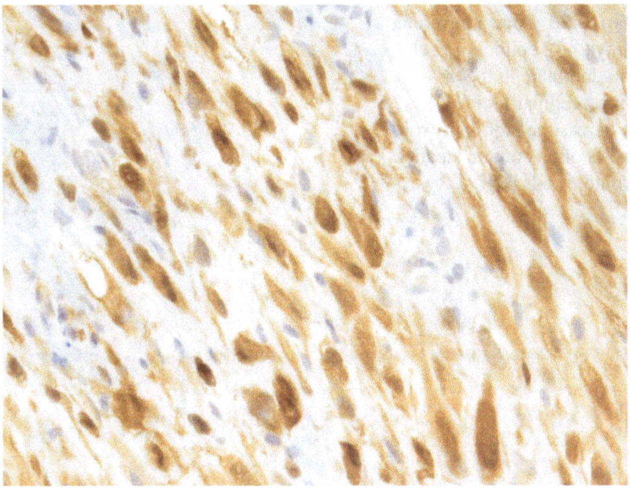

Fig. 6.25 PGP 9.5 is expressed by myxoid and cellular forms. There is nuclear and cytoplasmic staining

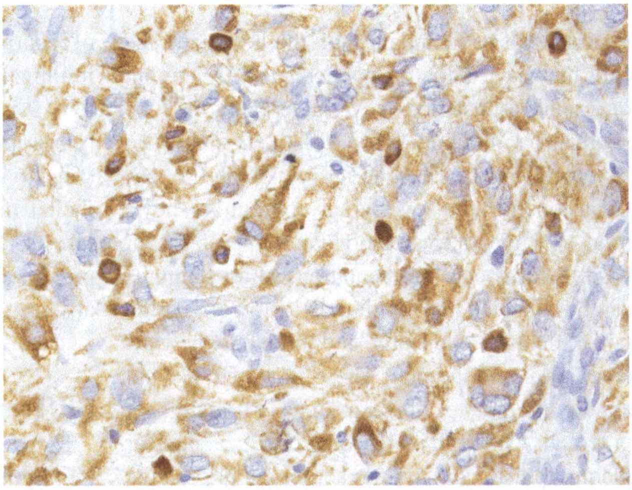

Fig. 6.26 NKI/C3, a lysosomal marker is expressed in a granular cytoplasmic pattern in neurothekeoma

myxoid forms of neurofibroma (NF), and angiomyxoma. NF is composed of cells with slender wavy nuclei, usually smaller and with less distinct cytoplasm than those of NTK. NF also contains axons (identified by special stains), and usually has a growth pattern readily identifiable as NF. The more common cellular forms of NTK have a broader differential diagnosis, including melanocytic neoplasms such as epithelioid Spitz nevus, deep penetrating nevus, and fascicular forms of cellular blue nevi. The latter group stains strongly for S-100 protein in addition to Melan-A and HMB-45. Fibrohistiocytic lesions such as epithelioid cell histiocytoma, epithelioid fibrous histiocytoma (dermatofibroma), and juvenile xanthogranuloma can be problematic, particularly because of the overlapping expression of monocytic/histiocytic markers. These typically lack the nested appearance of NTK. The histologic features of cellular NTK including infiltrative growth between collagen fibers, characteristic cytologic features, and the use of a broad immunohistochemical panel should facilitate this discrimination. Variants of pilar leiomyoma can be excluded based on the characteristic cigar-shaped, bubbly nuclear features, eosinophilic fine fibrillary cytoplasm, and the syncytial arrangements of fascicles of spindle cells, connection with existing pilar muscles, and the strong expression of smooth muscle-specific actin and sometimes desmin. NTK with a nodular or plexiform pattern must be distinguished from plexiform fibrohistiocytic tumor, although some authors suggest these entities are related. While both may have multinucleated cells, PFT often has a more prominent population of giant cells with usually deep soft tissue and subcutaneous involvement. PFHT is more diffusely and strongly reactive for CD68. The markedly nested, epithelioid variants of NTK can also mimic adnexal neoplasms and metastatic carcinoma, and rarely epithelioid angiosarcoma. Therefore, the application of cytokeratin stains, other epithelial markers relevant to a metastatic workup, and CD31 could help to establish the right diagnosis.

Primary Cutaneous Neuroendocrine Carcinoma (Merkel Cell Carcinoma)

Definition, Classification, and Histogenesis

Primary cutaneous neuroendocrine carcinoma (PCNC; Merkel cell carcinoma) is a high-grade malignant epithelial neoplasm with overlapping ultrastructural, histochemical, and immunohistochemical features of neurons and other neural crest-derived cells, including expression of synaptic proteins located on membrane bound vesicles. These neoplasms were once believed to derive from neural crest precursors. The term "neuroendocrine," however, is a misnomer, as the neoplastic cells are epithelial in nature and most likely do not derive from neural crest. Neverthe less, the term is firmly entrenched in the pathology lexicon and is retained here. Likewise, while the neoplastic cells of PCNC share features with Merkel cells, there is little evidence for a direct histogenetic relationship between the two. As such, the conceptually more unifying term PCNC is preferred over Merkel cell carcinoma. The latter is retained for historical purposes and familiarity. Recent investigations have identified a polyomavirus that appears to have an etiologic role in a major subset of these malignancies.

Clinical

PCNC occurs in late adulthood and is virtually nonexistent in children or young adults. The neoplasm is more prevalent in Caucasian males. Although this neoplasm may occur at any site, the head and neck, extremities, and buttocks are usual sites. Noncutaneous sites including nasal or oropharynx, vagina, or salivary glands may be affected. Typically, the cutaneous malignancy is a rapidly growing pink, red, or violaceous dome-shaped nodule. The overlying epidermis may be ulcerated. PCNC is often an aggressive malignancy associated with a protracted course, metastasis, and death. The 10-year survival rate is around 50%. Spontaneous regression is rare. Survival is best correlated with clinical staging.

Histopathology

PCNC involves the dermis, subcutaneous fat, or both, and commonly extends into fascia and muscle (Figs. 6.27–6.31). At scanning magnification, lesions may be circumscribed and nodular, or diffusely infiltrative. Various growth patterns exist within the mass including sheet-like, nested, and trabecular architecture. Epidermal involvement is less common (Figs. 6.29 and 6.32).The neoplastic cells are often monomorphic. There are two common appearances. In one type, the cells have small, round to oval nuclei about 2–3 times larger than mature lymphocytes, and resemble small cell carcinoma of the lung. Crush artifact is typical in this group. In other lesions, the neoplastic cells have enlarged round nuclei with fine nuclear chromatin, inconspicuous nucleoli, and distinct nuclear membranes (Fig. 6.33). The cytoplasm in both types is scant and nuclei are closely opposed. Mitotic figures and individual apoptotic cells are abundant. Large areas of necrosis are common, and there may be fibrosis and increased vascularity in the adjacent stroma. Rosette-like structures can occur, but true

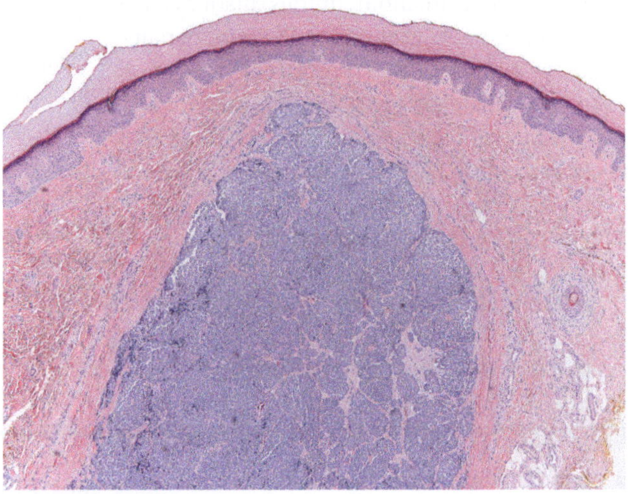

Fig. 6.27 Primary cutaneous neuroendocrine carcinoma: a circumscribed mass of neoplastic cells in the dermis

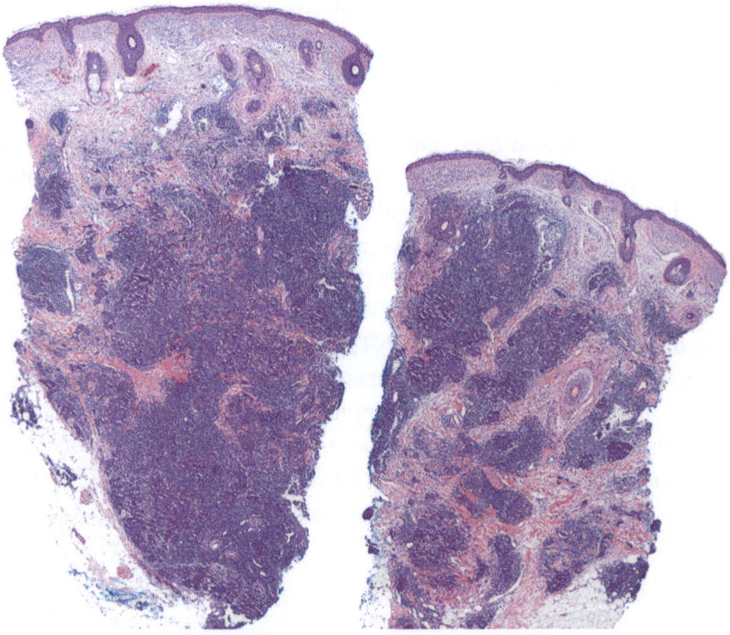

Fig. 6.28 Primary cutaneous neuroendocrine carcinoma: commonly this malignancy forms a highly infiltrative mass that occupies most of the dermis

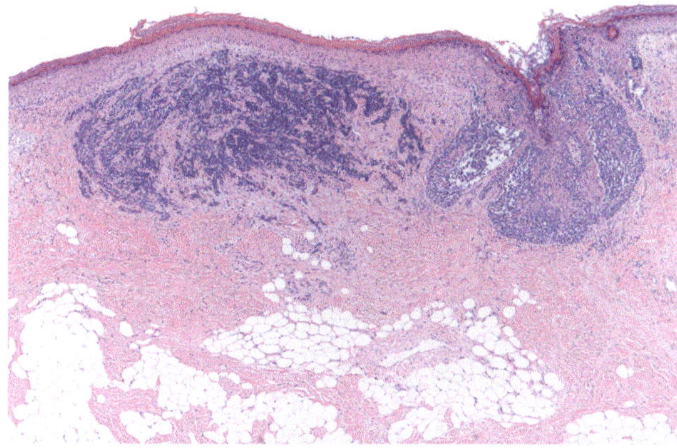

Fig. 6.29 Primary cutaneous neuroendocrine carcinoma: small clusters of malignant cells in the superficial dermis (*left*). A separate focus of epidermal involvement at the dermal–epidermal junction mimics superficial basal cell carcinoma. Intraepidermal upward spread of individual cells is present

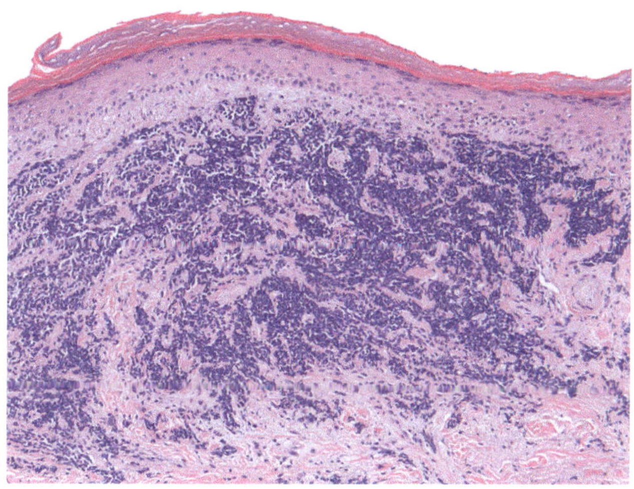

Fig. 6.30 Primary cutaneous neuroendocrine carcinoma: neoplastic cells with very scant cytoplasm. Most cells are individually inseparable because of high nuclear to cytoplasmic ratios

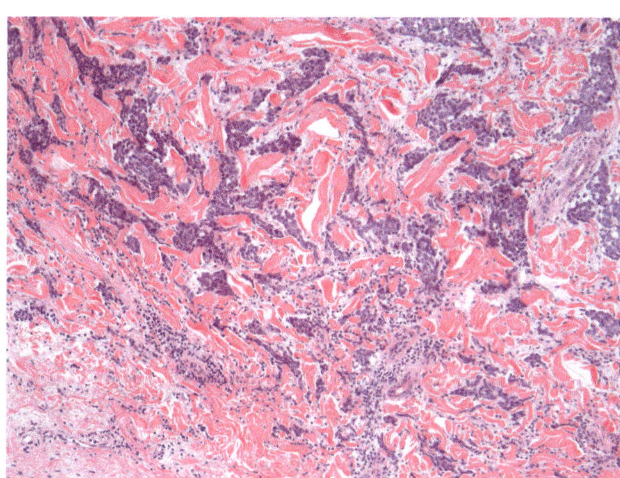

Fig. 6.31 Primary cutaneous neuroendocrine carcinoma: trabecular pattern with infiltrative nests and cords of neoplastic cells

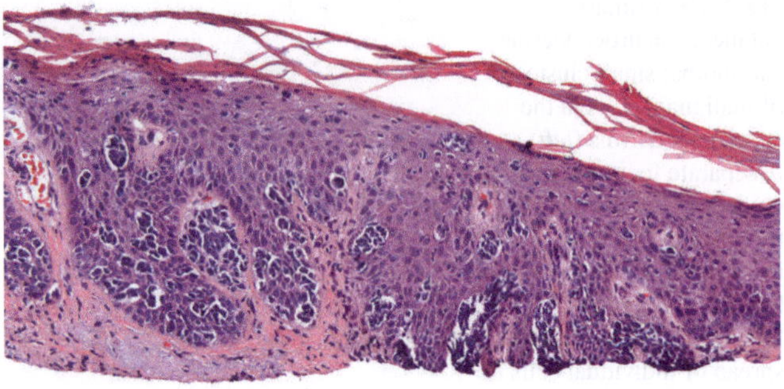

Fig. 6.32 Primary cutaneous neuroendocrine carcinoma: intraepidermal pagetoid spread mimics melanoma

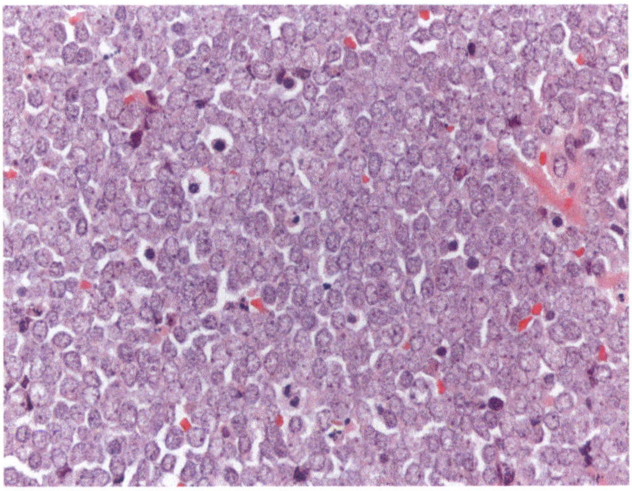

Fig. 6.33 Primary cutaneous neuroendocrine carcinoma: in well-preserved biopsies, the neoplastic cells have large monotonous nuclei, coarse chromatin, and indiscernible cytoplasm. Mitoses and apoptotic cells are prominent

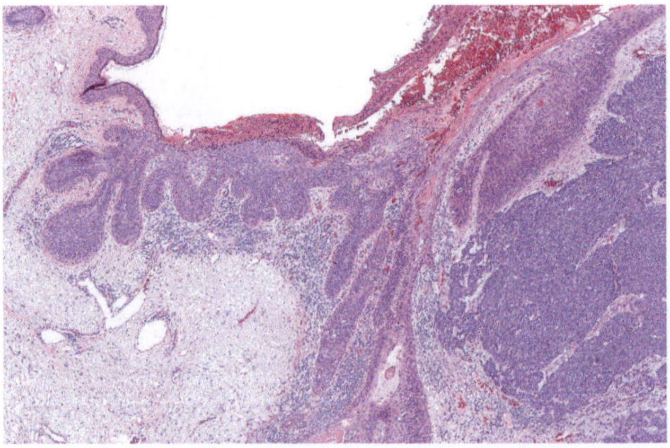

Fig. 6.34 Primary cutaneous neuroendocrine carcinoma: rarely the neoplasm arises in association with squamous cell carcinoma in situ. These forms often lack evidence of Merkel cell polyoma virus

rosettes are absent. Epidermotropism with pagetoid spread may raise consideration of a poorly differentiated squamous cell carcinoma or melanoma. Lymphocytes may be present mimicking lymphoepithelioma-like carcinoma. Importantly, some PCNC are associated with adjacent squamous cell carcinoma in situ or invasive squamous cell carcinoma (Fig. 6.34). In these neoplasms, the nuclei may show more variability in size and shape, coarse chromatin, and subtle hints of cytoplasm. PCNC arising in association with squamous neoplasms do not appear to be associated with polyoma virus.

Immunohistochemically, there is membranous and a characteristic paranuclear "dot-like" expression pattern with antibodies against low molecular weight cytokeratins and cytokeratin (CK) 20 (Fig. 6.35). This corresponds to paranuclear globular accumulations of intermediate filaments, visible by electron microscopy (Fig. 6.36). The cells also express epithelial membrane antigen. CK7 is less frequently present, and staining may be observed alone, or in conjunction with CK20. CK5/6 may be observed in PCNC, which arise in association with squamous cell carcinoma. There is expression of various neuroendocrine markers, including synaptophysin and chromogranin (Fig. 6.37a, b). Synaptophysin tends to be more sensitive, but either may show only weak or variable reactivity. PCNC also expresses neuron-specific enolase, neural filaments, and CD56 (Fig. 6.38). S-100 protein is negative. Like Ewing's sarcoma/PNET, CD99 and Fli-1 are often positive in PCNC. A subset stains for terminal deoxynucleotidyl

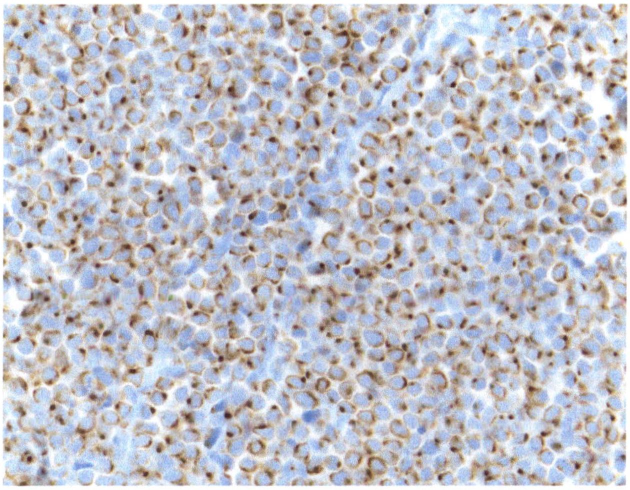

Fig. 6.35 Cytokeratin 20 is expressed by most cells in the majority of primary cutaneous neuroendocrine carcinomas. Characteristically, there is paranuclear dot-like expression but membranous staining may also be observed. In most cases cytokeratin 7 is negative

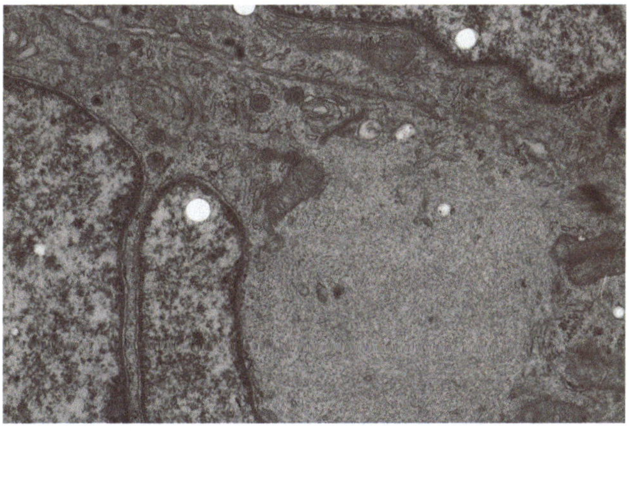

Fig. 6.36 Ultrastructural evaluation of primary cutaneous neuroendocrine carcinoma shows electron-dense secretory granules resembling those located near nerve synapses

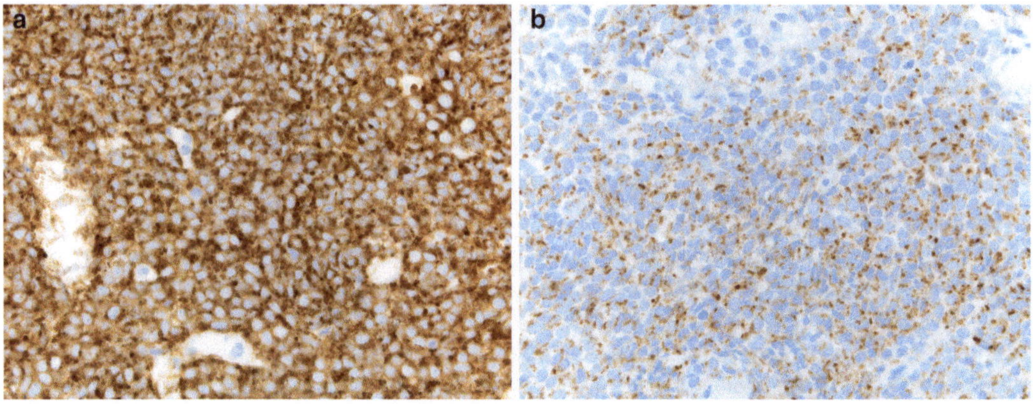

Fig. 6.37 (**a**) Synaptophysin expression is usually strong and diffuse. (**b**) Chromogranin expression is often variable and patchy

Fig. 6.38 Neuron-specific enolase expression is often diffuse

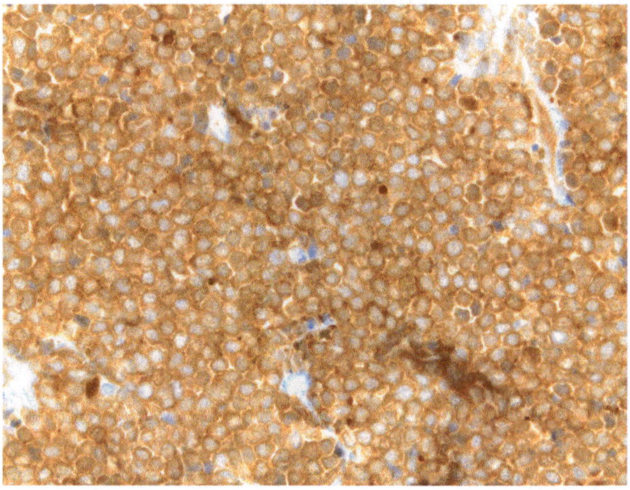

transferase (TdT), an important consideration in the distinction from acute lymphoblastic leukemia. Merkel cell polyomavirus may be detected by immunohistochemistry or molecular methods, a finding which could yield important diagnostic information if other immunostains are equivocal. It remains to be determined whether identification of this virus holds valuable prognostic information. Likewise, the expression of p63 has been implicated correlating with the prognosis.

Differential Diagnosis

Once epithelial differentiation is confirmed, the main diagnostic consideration is excluding cutaneous metastasis of visceral small cell carcinoma, particularly of pulmonary origin considering the common presentation of PCNC in older age. While this distinction requires close clinical correlation and imaging studies, immunohistochemistry is helpful. CK20 expression, combined with the absence of CK7 and thyroid transcription factor-1 (TTF-1) expression strongly favors PCNC. CK7 expression alone, however, provides only limited value, as positive staining may be observed in both PCNC and pulmonary small cell carcinoma. Importantly, detection of the polyoma virus also appears to be specific to PCNC. Small cell melanoma is excluded by negative reactivity for S-100 protein and other melanocytic markers. Acute lymphoblastic lymphoma, rhabdomyosarcoma, neuroblastoma, poorly differentiated eccrine carcinoma, and PNET/Ewing sarcoma must also be excluded. In general, these neoplasms are negative for CK20, and, in the former two, show appropriate evidence of hematopoietic or muscle differentiation. Refer to differential diagnostic Table A.4 of small, round blue cell tumors in Appendix.

Neurofollicular Hamartoma

Definition, Classification, and Histogenesis

Neurofollicular hamartoma (NFH) is an uncommon, benign hamartoma of epithelial and stromal cells. The etiologic nature of NFH is debated. Some authors consider these as a morphologic variant of fibrofolliculoma or trichodiscoma. Some cases may represent a pure coincidence of common neurofibroma associated with pilosebaceous units of glabrous skin. Convincing evidence of Schwann cell differentiation is lacking.

Clinical

Classically NFH presents a facial skin-colored papule. The skin on the nose or nasolabial fold is often affected. Lesions are asymptomatic and may resemble intradermal nevus or fibrous papule.

Histopathology

Fascicles of spindle cells occupy the superficial and deep dermis (Fig. 6.39). The spindle cells surround irregular or dilated hair follicles with large sebaceous glands (Figs. 6.40 and 6.41). The follicular epithelium may have an irregular appearance with cords and strands of epithelial cells extending into the dermis. There may be myxoid change. The spindle cells are small and uniform, resembling cells of intradermal nevus or neurofibroma (Figs. 6.42 and 6.43), but are positive for CD34 and negative for S-100 protein, suggesting fibrocytic rather than melanocytic or Schwann cell lineage. Scattered S-100 positive dendritic cells may be present.

Differential Diagnosis

NFH should be distinguished from neurofibroma, neurotized intradermal nevus, dermatofibroma, and benign fibrous papule. Neurofibroma is often more circumscribed in appearance and has a fine fibrillar stroma. Neurofibroma is partially composed of Schwann cells and therefore shows

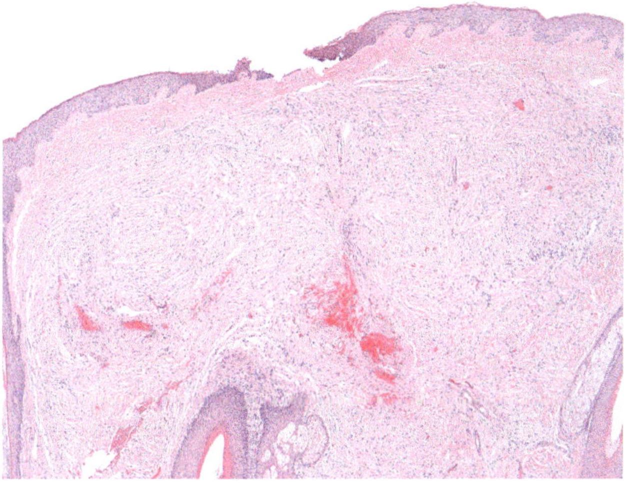

Fig. 6.39 Neurofollicular hamartoma: a circumscribed spindle cell proliferation in the dermis is present between hair follicles and is separated from the epidermis

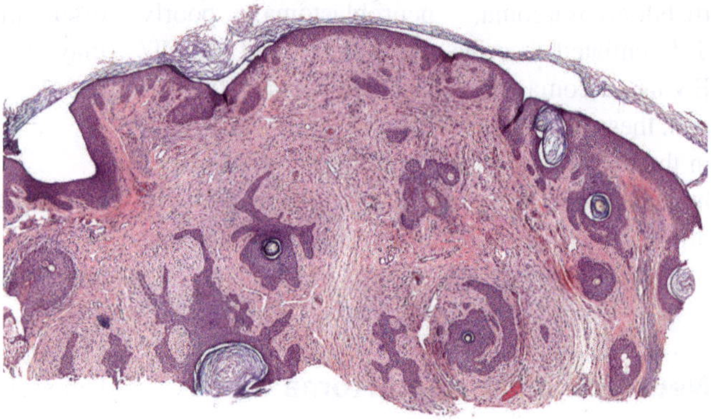

Fig. 6.40 Neurofollicular hamartoma: dermal spindle cells surround multiple hair follicles. The latter shows irregular projections of epithelium. These features are otherwise characteristic of the fibrofolliculoma/trichodiscoma family of hamartomas

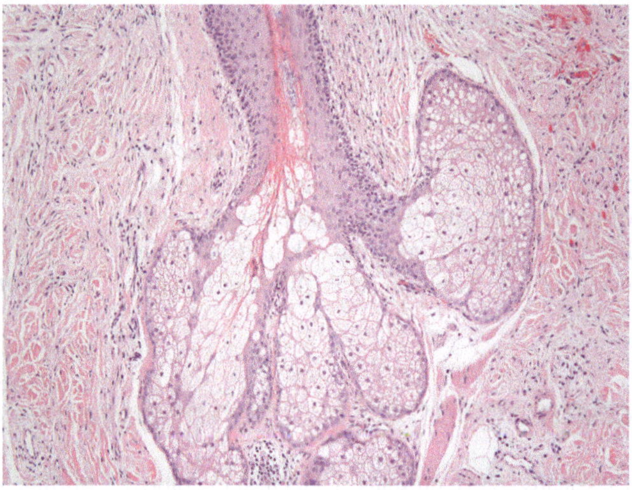

Fig. 6.41 Neurofollicular hamartoma: the spindle cells are closely arranged around folliculo-sebaceous units, resembling the growth of neurotized melanocytic nevi. In contrast to nevi, the cells tend to entrap collagen fibers

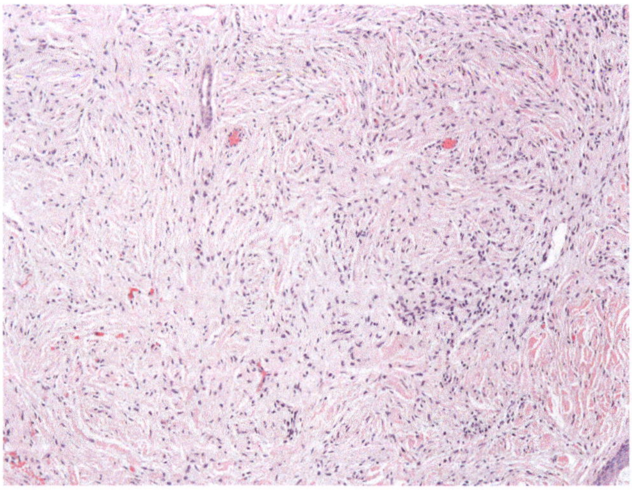

Fig. 6.42 Neurofollicular hamartoma: the spindle cells have a slightly whorled appearance

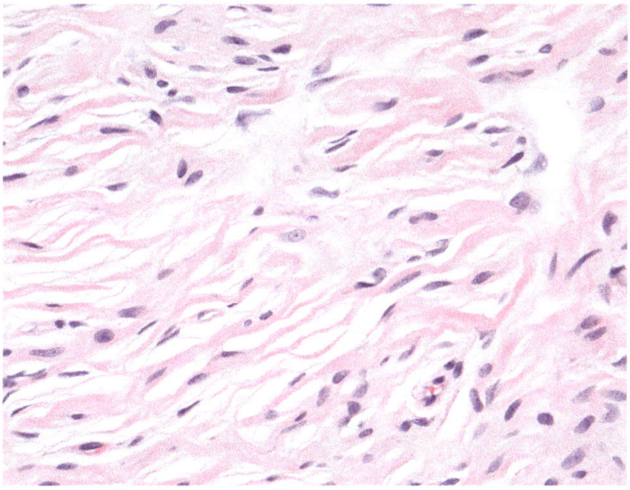

Fig. 6.43 Neurofollicular hamartoma: the spindle cells have bland slender nuclei. In these cases, S-100 protein expression is negative, distinguishing from the Schwann cells of neurofibroma or melanocytic cells

expression of S-100 protein. A neurotized melanocytic nevus will often have nests of epithelioid cells recognizable as melanocytic in nature. If absent, expression of S-100 protein and Melan-A identifies the lesion as melanocytic. Of note, intradermal nevus will often show prominent growth along adnexal structures but usually the adnexal are not hyperplastic. Dermatofibroma consists of spindle cells with admixed lymphocytes with or without vacuolated histiocytes. Often the stroma is sclerotic. Although follicular hyperplasia may be present, the intervening epidermis is often acanthotic with basilar hyperpigmentation. DF often has a prominent Grenz zone, whereas in NFH the spindle cells are localized immediately adjacent to the adnexal. Fibrous papule is less cellular than NFH with a more sclerotic appearing stroma, stellate or multinucleated stromal cells, and dilated vessels.

Additional Reading

Neurothekeoma

Fetsch JF, Laskin WB, Hallman JR, Lupton GP, Miettinen M. Neurothekeoma: an analysis of 178 tumors with detailed immunohistochemical data and long-term patient follow-up information. Am J Surg Pathol. 2007;31:1103–14.

Hornick JL, Fletcher CD. Cellular neurothekeoma: detailed characterization in a series of 133 cases. Am J Surg Pathol. 2007;31:329–40.

Plaza JA, Torres-Cabala C, Evans H, Diwan AH, Prieto VG. Immunohistochemical expression of S100A6 in cellular neurothekeoma: clinicopathologic and immunohistochemical analysis of 31 cases. Am J Dermatopathol. 2009;31:419–22.

Primary Cutaneous Neuroendocrine Carcinoma

Busam KJ, Jungbluth AA, Rekthman N, Coit D, Pulitzer M, Bini J, et al. Merkel cell polyomavirus expression in merkel cell carcinomas and its absence in combined tumors and pulmonary neuroendocrine carcinomas. Am J Surg Pathol. 2009;33:1378–85.

Duncavage EJ, Le BM, Wang D, Pfeifer JD. Merkel cell polyomavirus: a specific marker for Merkel cell carcinoma in histologically similar tumors. Am J Surg Pathol. 2009;33:1771–7.

Neurofollicular Hamartoma

Barr RJ, Goodman MM. Neurofollicular hamartoma: a light microscopy and immunohistochemical study. J Cutan Pathol. 1989;16:336–41.

Sangueza OP, Requena L. Neurofollicular hamartoma: a new histogenetic interpretation. Am J Dermatopathol. 1994;16:150–4.

Cutaneous Neuroblastic and Ganglion Cell Proliferations

7

Keywords
Cutaneous neuroblastic and ganglionic tumors • Definition • Classification, Histogenesis • Diagnostic features • Differential diagnosis neuroblastoma • Ganglioneuroma • Ganglion cell choristoma

Neuroblastoma

Definition, Classification, and Histogenesis

Neuroblastoma is a malignant neoplasm of neural crest lineage, most often arising in the adrenal medulla, paraganglia, or sympathetic chain. Cutaneous neuroblastoma usually represents metastasis from a visceral primary. However, rare cutaneous neuroblastoma may develop de novo without an identifiable visceral tumor, possibly from heterotopic neural crest cells. Neuroblastoma represents the most primitive form in a family of neoplasms, which includes ganglioneuroma at the opposite, mature end of the spectrum.

Clinical Findings

Cutaneous neuroblastoma usually appears as multiple blue or purple papules and nodules. This appearance is similar to the "blueberry muffin" lesions of extramedullary hematopoiesis of congenital rubella syndrome. The lesions blanch with pressure. Serum and urine catecholamines may be increased. Spontaneous regression may occur. Primary cutaneous neuroblastoma is exceedingly rare. It is usually present in adults as rapidly growing dermal nodules. These are highly aggressive neoplasms with an almost invariably fatal outcome.

Histologic Features

There is often an ill-defined, infiltrative proliferation of irregular nests, cords, or sheets (Fig. 7.1). The lesional cells of neuroblastoma have small round nuclei with fine chromatin and scant cytoplasm (Fig. 7.2a, b). Neuroblastomas are therefore among the so-called small round blue cell tumors. Homer Wright rosettes are common, and consist of concentric rings of nuclei with a distinct anuclear center of finely fibrillar material resembling neuropil (Fig. 7.3a, b). These structures are pathognomonic of neuroblastoma. Brisk mitotic activity, necrosis, and hemorrhage are common. Partial maturation typified by the presence of ganglion cells and/or a schwannian stroma may be seen.

The immunophenotypic expression appears to correlate with the stage of maturation. Primitive forms may react with neuron-specific enolase, synaptophysin, neural filaments, and chromogranin (Fig. 7.4). The more differentiated forms of neuroblastoma may also stain for S-100 protein.

Z. Argenyi and C.H. Jokinen (eds.), *Cutaneous Neural Neoplasms*, Current Clinical Pathology,
DOI 10.1007/978-1-60327-582-8_7, © Springer Science+Business Media, LLC 2011

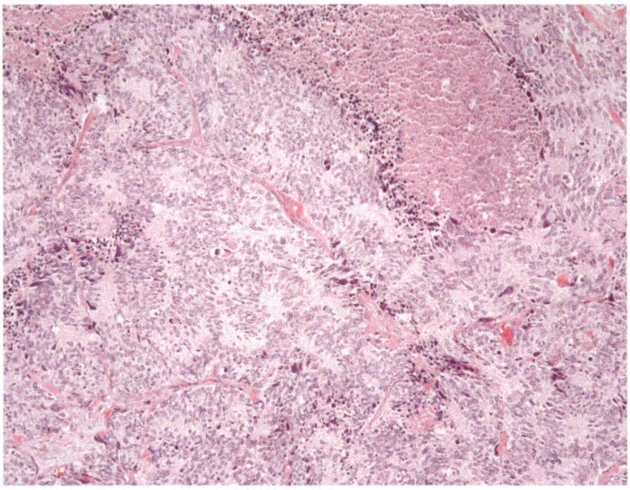

Fig. 7.1 Cutaneous neuroblastoma: sheets of primitive epithelioid cells with large areas of necrosis

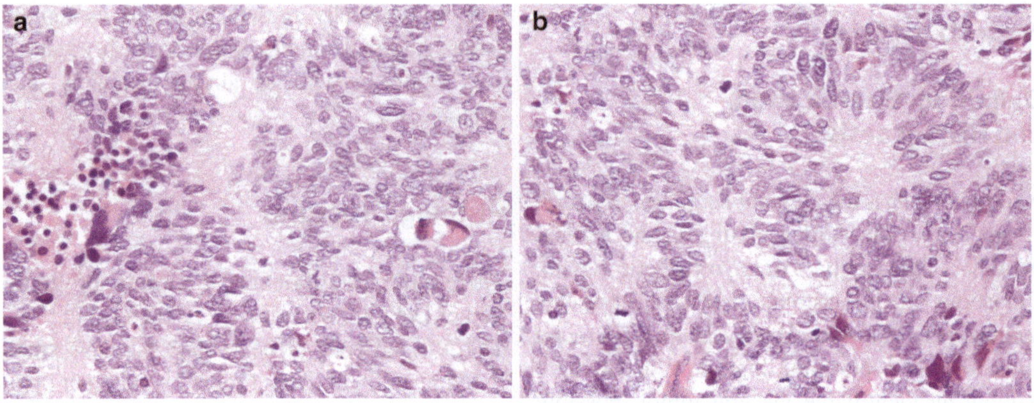

Fig. 7.2 Cutaneous neuroblastoma: (**a**) the lesional cells have monotonous ovoid nuclei with fine chromatin. Individual necrotic cells are present. (**b**) Characteristic Homer Wright rosettes with peripheral palisades of nuclei and central cores of cytoplasmic processes and stroma

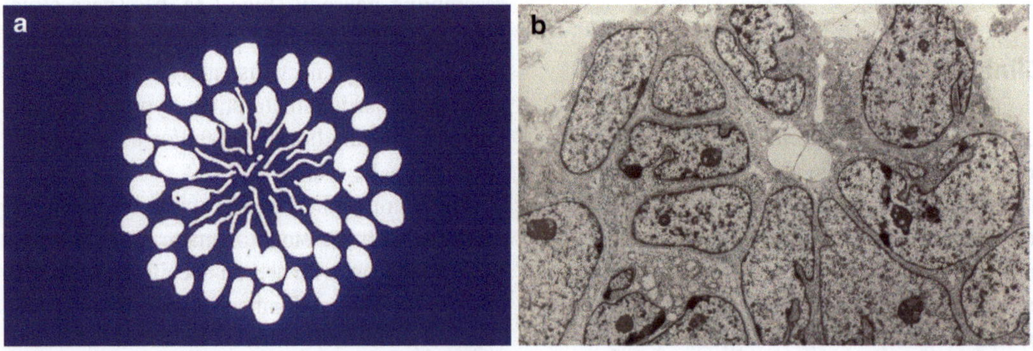

Fig. 7.3 (**a**) Schematic representation of *true* (*Homer Wright*) *rosette* common to neuroblastoma. There is a central core of cytoplasmic processes (artwork by ZA). (**b**) Corresponding ultrastructural examination shows multiple cytoplasmic processes directed toward the center of the rosette. The cells have highly irregular nuclei and little cytoplasm

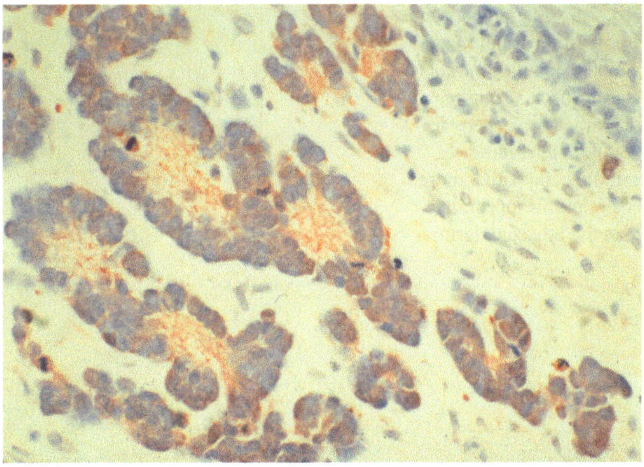

Fig. 7.4 Neuron-specific enolase immunostain highlights the scant cytoplasm and central arrays of cytoplasmic processes in the centers of the rosettes

Differential Diagnosis

Metastatic neuroblastoma may be confused with the other small, round, blue cell tumors, especially if rosette-like structures are present. However, true Homer Wright rosettes are not characteristic of any of the following entities: primary neuroendocrine carcinoma of the skin (Merkel cell carcinoma), metastatic small cell carcinoma of the lung, extraskeletal Ewing's sarcoma, embryonal rhabdomyosarcoma, poorly differentiated eccrine carcinoma, small cell malignant melanoma, and precursor B-cell lymphoblastic lymphoma. As discussed under primary neuroendocrine carcinoma of the skin, immunohistochemistry and electron microscopy have an important role in rendering the correct diagnosis. Please refer to the differential diagnostic chart of small, round, blue cell tumors in Table A.4 in Appendix.

Ganglioneuroma

Definition, Classification, and Histogenesis

Cutaneous ganglioneuroma is a rare neoplasm composed of mature ganglion cells and Schwann cells. In viscera, ganglioneuroma is considered a mature form of the neuroblastoma family of neoplasms. The ganglion cells represent the mature "cellular" element, while the Schwann cells comprise the mature "stromal" population. In the skin, ganglioneuromas may represent maturation of metastatic neuroblastoma. Nevertheless, most cutaneous ganglioneuromas develop without evidence of an underlying neuroblastoma. These may represent abnormal migration of neural crest cells during development.

Clinical

Ganglioneuroma may present at any anatomic site, but most reported cases arise on the proximal extremities and trunk. These affect newborns, children, and adults. Lesions are often flesh-colored papules and asymptomatic.

Histopathology

Ganglioneuroma is a well-circumscribed dermal mass that lacks encapsulation (Fig. 7.5). Most of the mass is composed of uniform spindle cells with wavy buckled nuclei, otherwise typical of Schwann cells. Admixed is a smaller population of ganglion cells. Ganglion cells are large polygonal cells with an eccentric large round nucleus, fine chromatin, and prominent single nucleolus (Fig. 7.6). Nissl substance may be present. Ganglion cells are positive for synaptophysin, GFAP, PGP 9.5, neuron-specific enolase (Figs. 7.7–7.9), and neurofilaments. Data are conflicting regarding expression of S-100 protein, which is usually negative, but may be variable

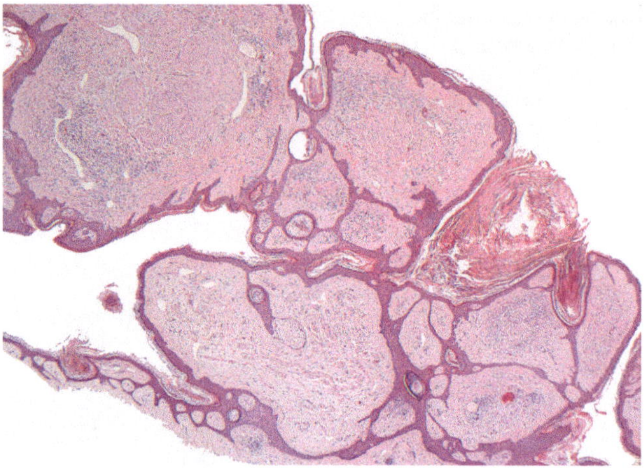

Fig. 7.5 Ganglioneuroma: a polypoid dermal mass which resembles intradermal nevus at scanning magnification. There are nodular aggregates of spindle cells with a more eosinophilic appearance than the adjacent dermis

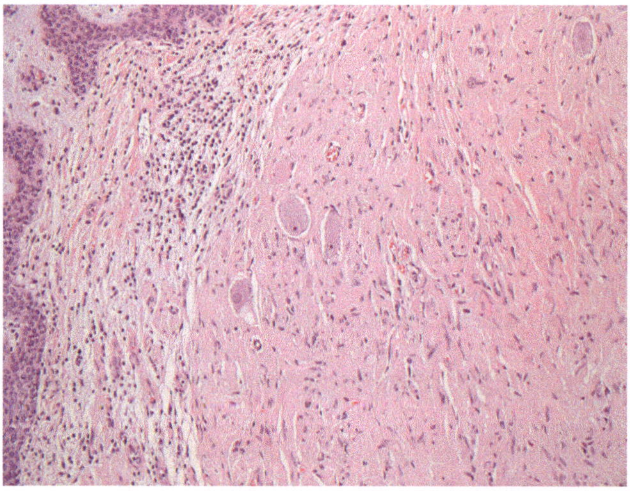

Fig. 7.6 Ganglioneuroma: the eosinophilic aggregates are composed of Schwann cells with uniform slender nuclei, and abundant axons which are highlighted by immunohistochemistry. Admixed are ganglion cells with large round nuclei, a single macronucleolus, and abundant cytoplasm. Retraction artifact around the ganglion cells is typical

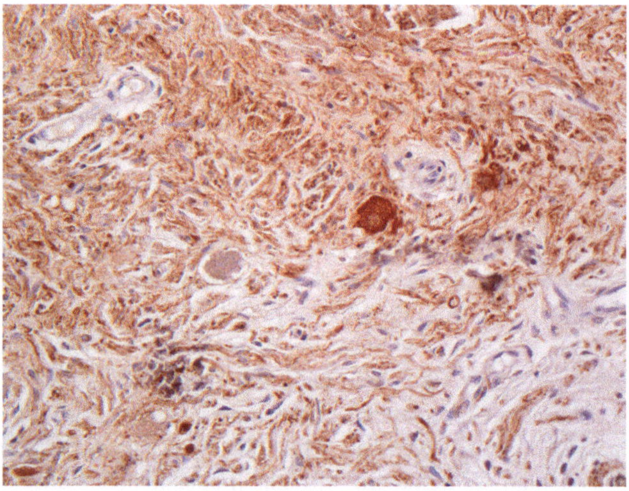

Fig. 7.7 Neuron-specific enolase: there is staining of the ganglion cells and stroma. Ganglion cells may also express synaptophysin and GFAP

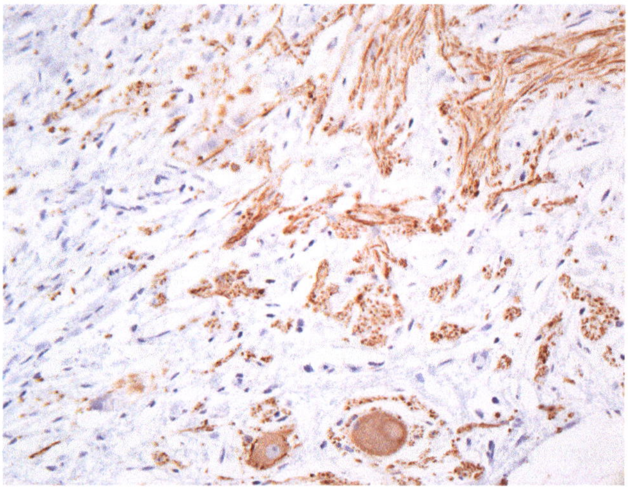

Fig. 7.8 Neurofilaments immunostain: there is staining of the ganglion cells and axons present in the adjacent stroma

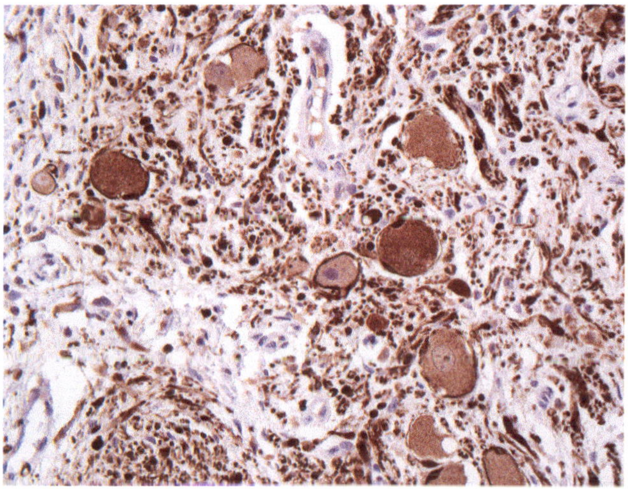

Fig. 7.9 S-100 protein expression is positive in the ganglion cells and the Schwann cells in the nearby stroma. The ganglion cells however show variable staining with this marker and negative staining should not preclude a diagnosis

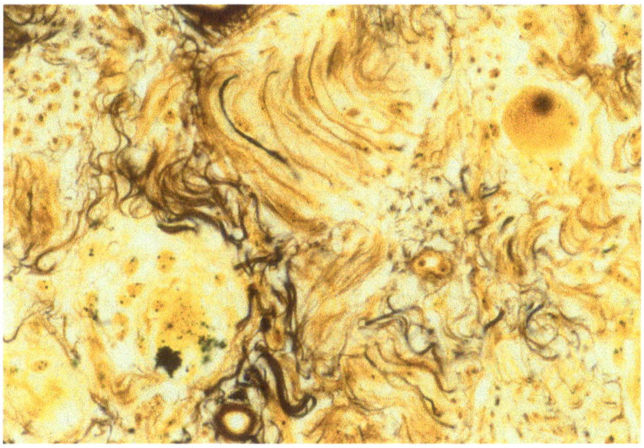

Fig. 7.10 Silver impregnation of ganglioneuroma showing numerous axons, black linear structures, adjacent to ganglion cells

and weak. The Schwann cells are uniformly and strongly positive for S-100 protein. The axons can also be demonstrated by conventional silver stain (Fig. 7.10).

Differential Diagnosis

The combination of ganglion cells and Schwann cells is a unique finding. Ganglion cell choristoma (GCC) lacks the schwannian stroma of ganglioneuroma. The large polygonal ganglion cells should be distinguished from melanocytic neoplasms including Spitz nevus, combined nevus, and spitzoid melanoma. These proliferations, being melanocytic in nature, express Melan-A. An obvious junctional component is also diagnostic of a melanocytic nevus when present. Pure dermal Spitz nevi are composed of epithelioid cells, which are somewhat smaller and rounder than the typical large and polygonal ganglion cells. Additionally, Spitz nevi lack a Schwann cell-rich stroma. Epithelioid fibrous histiocytoma and reticulohistiocytoma may also be considered. However, these cells usually lack nucleoli and are typically much smaller than the usual ganglion cell. These are also distinguished by the reactivity for CD163 or factor XIIIa and the lack of typical markers of ganglion cells.

Ganglion Cell Choristoma

Definition, Classification, and Histogenesis

GCC is exceedingly rare, and possibly related to ganglioneuroma. In contrast to the latter, GCC is composed only of ganglion cells without an associated Schwannian stroma. The histogenesis is unknown.

Clinical

No diagnostic clinical descriptions are available as very few cases are reported.

Histopathology

GCC is a dermal mass composed of clusters of ganglion cells, similar to those of normal tissues or ganglioneuroma. Unlike ganglioneuroma, GCC lacks schwannian stroma.

Differential Diagnosis

GCC is distinguished from ganglioneuroma by the lack of a schwannian stroma. The ganglion cells themselves may resemble melanocytes or epithelioid histiocytes. A complete description of ganglion cells can be found in the preceding section.

Additional Reading

Furmanczyk PS, Hughes SR, Walsh JS, Bass J, McFarlane JR, Argenyi ZB. Cutaneous ganglioneuroma associated with overlying hyperkeratotic epidermal changes: a report of 2 cases. Am J Dermatopathol. 2008;30:600–3.

Wallace CA, Hallman JR, Sangueza OP. Primary cutaneous ganglioneuroma: a report of two cases and literature review. Am J Dermatopathol. 2003;25:239–42.

Cutaneous Glial and Meningothelial Proliferations

8

Keywords
Cutaneous glial and meningothelial tumors • Definition • Classification • Histogenesis • Diagnostic features • Differential diagnosis • Heterotopic glial tissue • Meningioma • Meningocele • Encephalocele

Glial and meningothelial proliferations of the skin are rare. In this chapter, nasal glioma (glial heterotopia), meningocele, and cutaneous meningioma are discussed. As a group, these lesions represent a spectrum of abnormalities related to abnormal closure of the neural tube or abnormal migration of neural crest cells during development; therefore, semantically some of them are not considered true neoplasms, but as ectopic or heterotopic cell nests which can be the origin of a neoplastic proliferation.

Nasal Glioma (Heterotopic Glial Tissue)

Definition, Classification, and Histogenesis

Nasal glioma is a heterotopic mass of neuroglial tissue that results from herniation of brain into the nasal cavity and nasal skin. *Nasal glioma* is a misnomer, as this lesion is not a glial neoplasm like that of the central nervous system. The term is retained however for historical purposes and familiarity.

Clinical Findings

Nasal gliomas are solitary, firm, flesh-colored, or erythematous nodules. Most are congenital, although occasionally it may present in later life. They may appear clinically as hemangiomas. About 30% of nasal gliomas are intranasal, whereas 10% may have both extranasal and intranasal involvement. Cutaneous lesions are often present on the nasal bridge. Intranasal forms may exert pressure on adjacent structures. Encephaloceles, which histologically are identical to heterotopic glial tissue, communicate with the intracranial cavity. Therefore, radiologic imaging is performed prior to biopsy in order to prevent meningoencephalitis (Fig. 8.1).

Histopathology

Nasal glioma or heterotopic glial tissue is composed of the various cell types and stromal support system of mature brain tissue. It appears as a dermal or subcutaneous lobular mass, which at scanning magnification has an eosinophilic appearance (Fig. 8.2). The neuropil has a fine fibrillar and vacuolated appearance. Admixed blood vessels, fibrosis, and inflammation may be present. Within the stroma, there are scattered neurons admixed with various glial cells. Mature neurons are characterized by large, polygonal cell bodies, with large, eccentric round nuclei, and prominent nucleoli (Fig. 8.3a, b). The neurons contain Nissl substance, and have dendritic and axonal cytoplasmic extensions. The most

Z. Argenyi and C.H. Jokinen (eds.), *Cutaneous Neural Neoplasms*, Current Clinical Pathology,
DOI 10.1007/978-1-60327-582-8_8, © Springer Science+Business Media, LLC 2011

common glial cells are the mature astrocytes with a round nucleus, prominent nucleolus, and distinct nuclear membrane. There is often a halo around the cytoplasmic membrane. Fibrillary astrocytes have elongated eosinophilic processes, whereas gemistocytic astrocytes are polygonal, have brightly eosinophilic cytoplasm and peripherally displaced nuclei (Fig. 8.4a). Partial retention of the meningothelial lining may be present at the periphery. Ependymal cells or pigmented cells may also be identified. The neurons stain for neuron-specific enolase and synaptophysin. The axons react with antibodies to neural filaments and the glial tissue labels for antibodies to glial fibrillary acidic protein (GFAP) (Fig. 8.4b). If residual meningothelial lining is present it can be highlighted by EMA.

Differential Diagnosis

Nasal glioma is microscopically identical to encephalocele and radiologic imaging is required for distinction. Other diagnostic considerations

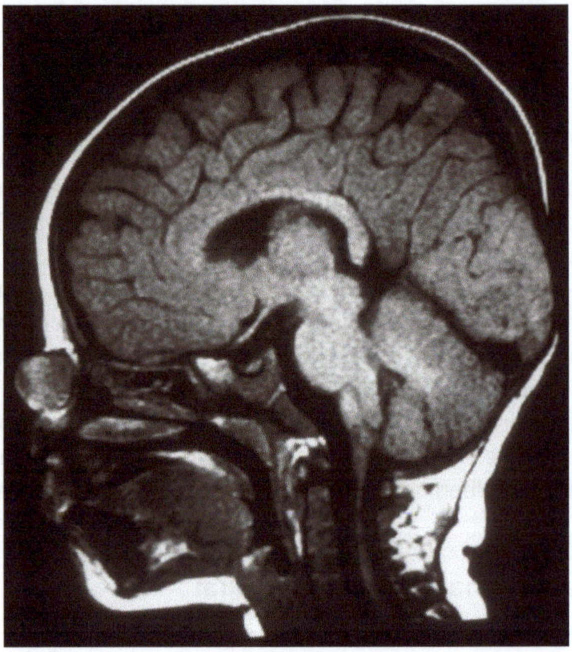

Fig. 8.1 Imaging study of nasal glioma shows a large polypoid mass of frontal cranium

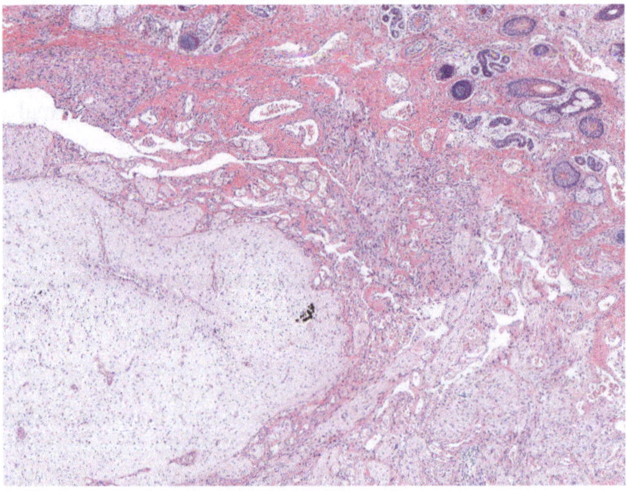

Fig. 8.2 Nasal glioma (heterotopic glial tissue): nasal mucosa with a multinodular mass and fibrosis

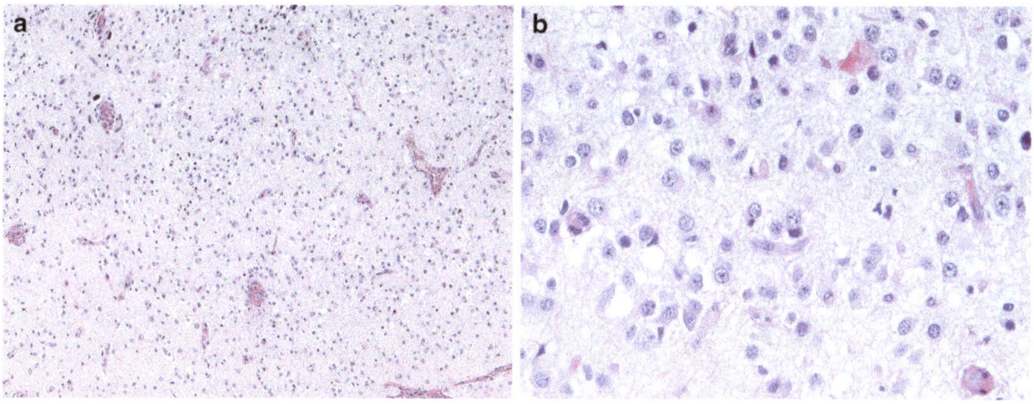

Fig. 8.3 (**a**) Nasal glioma: pale fibrillar neuroglial tissue with prominent vessels. (**b**) Nasal glioma: neurons with large round nuclei, fine chromatin, and eccentric eosinophilic cytoplasm are mixed with astrocytes and abundant neuropil

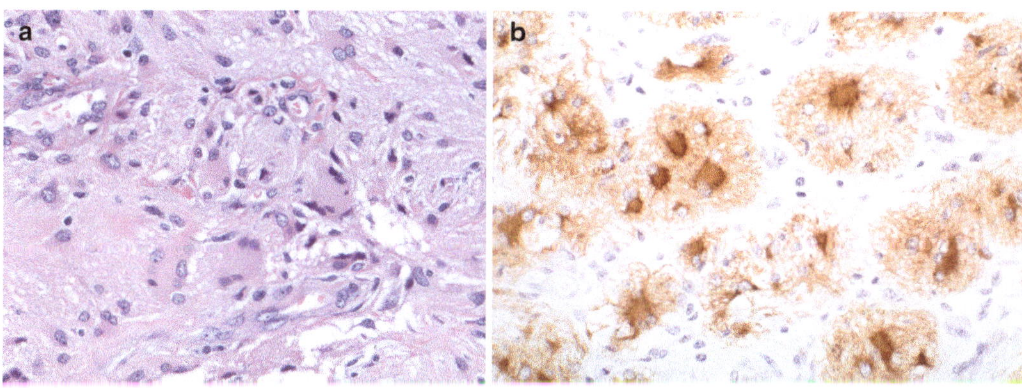

Fig. 8.4 (**a**) Nasal glioma: gemistocytic astrocytes have abundant dense eosinophilic cytoplasm. (**b**) GFAP immunostain highlights the delicate fibrillary glial network

include ganglioneuroma or dermoid cyst. Ganglioneuroma is distinguished by its Schwann cell-rich stroma that is diffusely positive for S-100 protein. Dermoid cysts contain other tissues including epithelium.

Cutaneous Meningioma

Definition, Classification, and Histogenesis

Meningioma is a neoplasm of meningothelial cells. Cutaneous meningioma most commonly represents a primary cutaneous neoplasm. These likely arise from precursor cells abnormally displaced to the skin during development. Cutaneous extension of a meningioma arising in the central nervous system may also occur including from the lining of the cranial nerves. These are typically associated with worse prognosis.

Clinical

The primary or congenital lesions usually follow the cranial or vertebral closure lines along the path of the cranial nerves. They are more common in newborns or in children and they follow a favorable biological course. Secondary lesions usually affect adults as cutaneous metastasis from underlying primary meningioma of the arachoidal lining of the cranium. This manifestation is extremely rare and heralds a poor prognosis.

Histopathology

Cutaneous meningioma usually present as an ill-defined subcutaneous or a dermal mass which shares cytologic features with rudimentary meningocele; however, cystic or pseudovascular spaces are not present. The lesional cells are mostly epithelioid or slightly spindled cells, with oval nuclei and vesicular chromatin (Figs. 8.5–8.7). The cells often form nests with a whorl-like pattern, otherwise characteristic of intracranial meningioma. Calcified papillary structures or psammoma bodies are common (Fig. 8.8). Mitotic figures are uncommon. In metastatic forms, however, pleomorphism and mitoses may be prominent. Immunohistochemically, the neoplastic cells are positive for epithelial membrane antigen and vimentin. Progesterone receptor is commonly positive in central nervous system forms, but additional studies are needed to assess its usefulness in cutaneous lesions. Rare expression of S-100 protein,

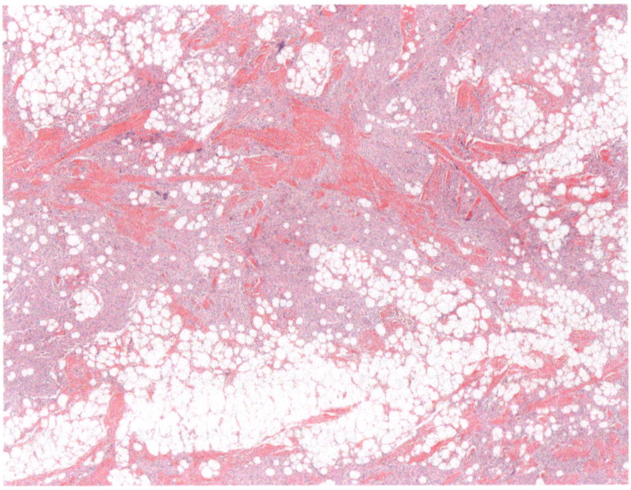

Fig. 8.5 Cutaneous meningioma: subcutaneous proliferation of nests and cords

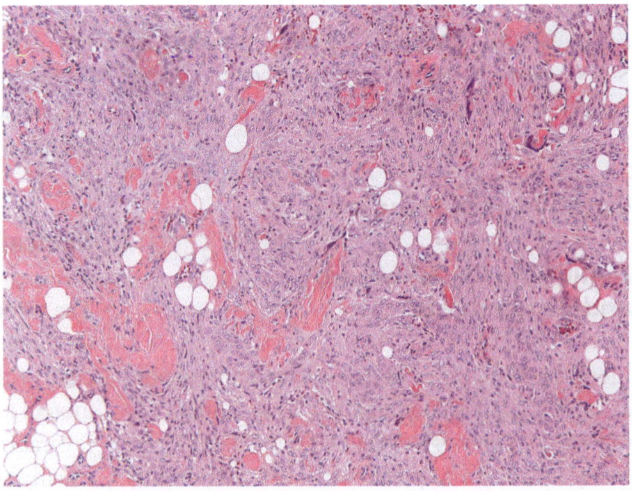

Fig. 8.6 Cutaneous meningioma: epithelioid cells form whorls within the nests

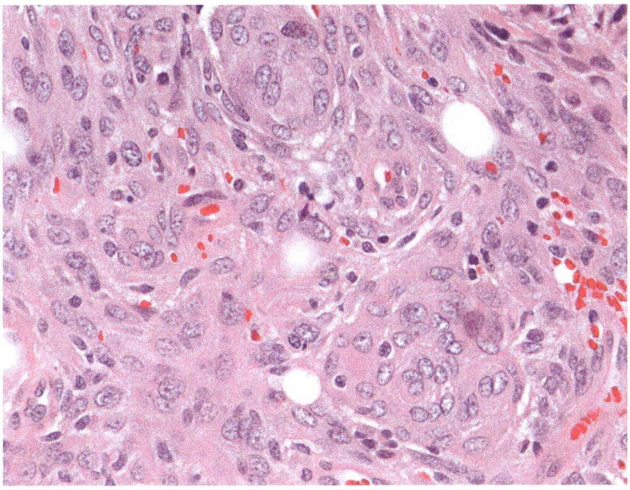

Fig. 8.7 Cutaneous meningioma: uniform round nuclei with vesicular chromatin and eosinophilic cytoplasm

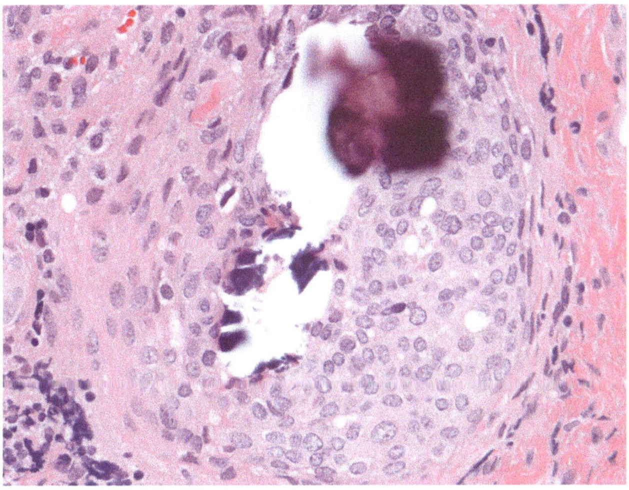

Fig. 8.8 Cutaneous meningioma: psammoma bodies are common

neuron-specific enolase, and cytokeratins are described but these markers are usually negative.

Differential Diagnosis

Meningioma may at first glance resemble a variety of more common cutaneous neoplasms. Epithelioid forms should be differentiated from cellular neurothekeoma, squamous cell carcinoma, or adnexal neoplasms. None of these other entities forms the typical nests with a whorled appearance common to meningioma. Among these, psammoma bodies are also highly suspicious for meningioma. Cellular neurothekeoma is negative for EMA. Furthermore, diffuse, strong cytokeratin expression favors carcinoma or an adnexal neoplasm. Spindled forms may resemble cellular blue nevus, which is distinguished by strong staining for Melan-A and S-100 protein.

Meningocele

Definition, Classification, and Histogenesis

Meningocele is a benign, nonproliferative heterotopia of meningothelial cells, which represents herniation of meningothelial tissue along faulty lines of closure during development.

Meningoceles can be further defined as "classical or rudimentary." In the classical variant, there is a well-established connection with the brain and its lining, whereas in rudimentary form there is no distinct connection present. When the meningothelial cells are associated with brain tissue (neurons, glia/neuropil), the term meningoencephalocele is applied.

Clinical

Rudimentary meningocele presents as soft flesh-colored papules and nodules along the lines of cranial closure on the scalp. Alopecia or abnormal hair growth may be observed on the overlying skin.

Histopathology

Rudimentary meningocele is a poorly defined deep dermal or subcutaneous mass (Fig. 8.9). Epithelioid or stellate cells with ovoid nuclei, fine chromatin, and eosinophilic cytoplasm infiltrate and dissect adjacent thickened collagen fibers (Figs. 8.10 and 8.11). These may form large cystic spaces that resemble ectatic blood vessels. Collagen bodies are often present and formed when hyalinized collagen fibers are completely

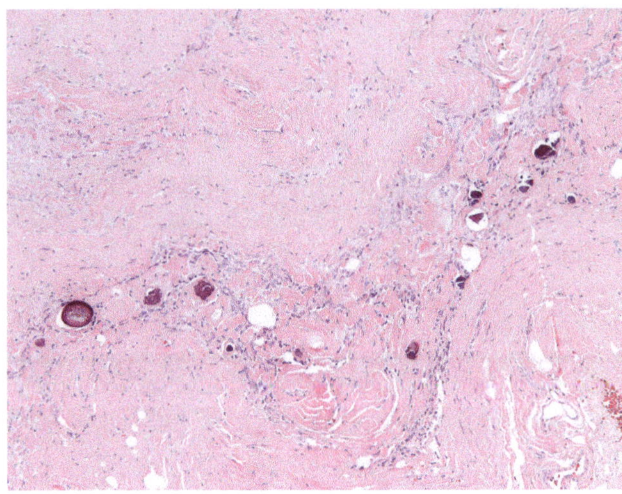

Fig. 8.9 Rudimentary meningocele: thin cords of meningothelial cells in a densely fibrous stroma. Numerous psammomatous calcifications are present

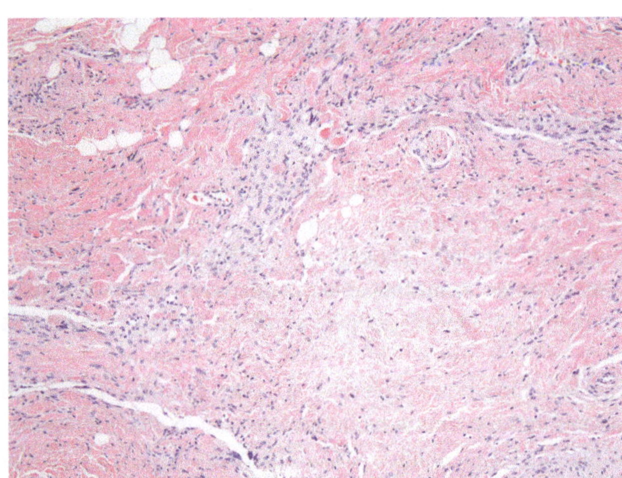

Fig. 8.10 Rudimentary meningocele: single cells and cords of epithelioid cells

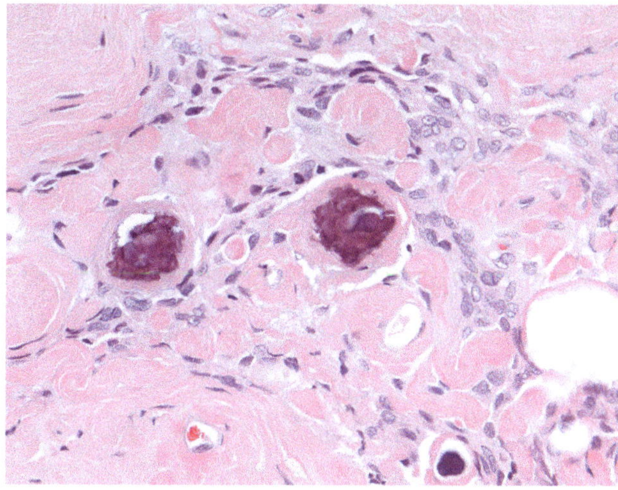

Fig. 8.11 Rudimentary meningocele: the cells have a cytologic appearance identical to those of meningioma

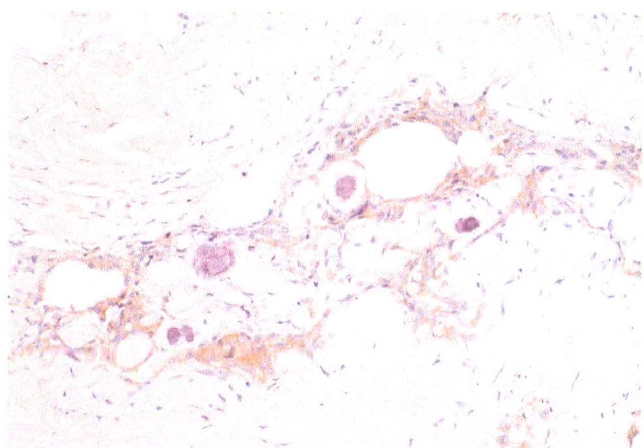

Fig. 8.12 Rudimentary meningocele: EMA immunostain delineates meningothelial cells within the fibrous stroma

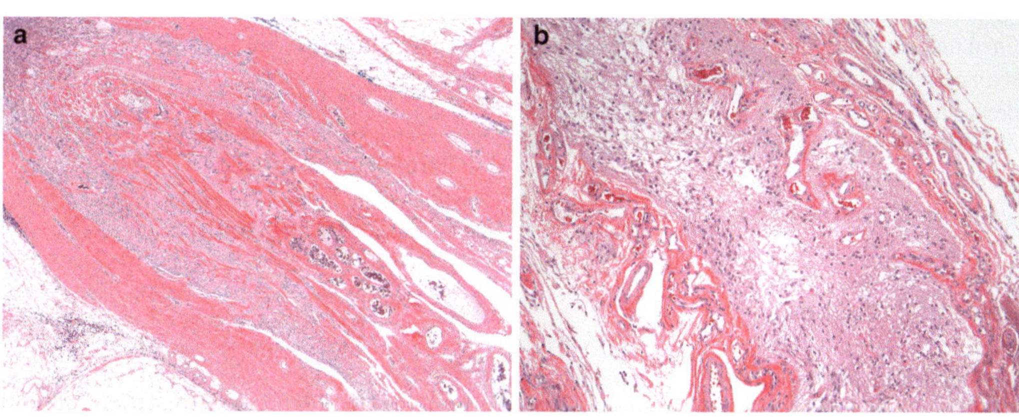

Fig. 8.13 (**a**) Meningoencephalocele: ectopic meningothelial cells and neuroglial tissue. (**b**) Meningoencephalocele: astrocytes, oligodendrocytes, and abundant neuropil

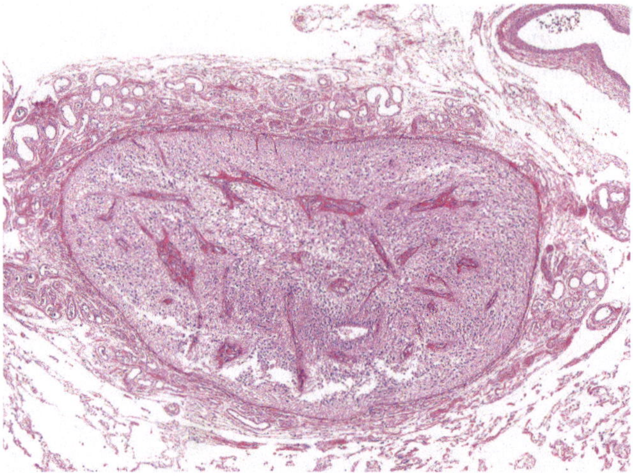

Fig. 8.14 Meningoencephalocele: nodule of ectopic brain tissue

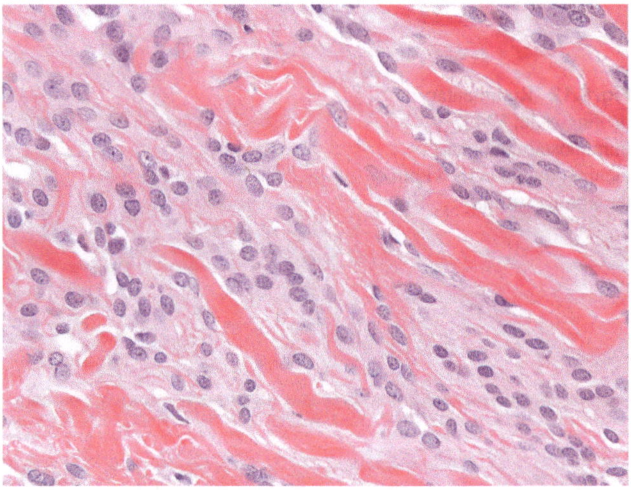

Fig. 8.15 Meningoencephalocele: cords of meningothelial cells

surrounded by meningothelial cells. Psammoma bodies with or without calcifications are common (Fig. 8.11). Classical meningoceles form a well-defined mass and lack the infiltrative and pseudovascular architecture. The meningothelial cells express EMA (Fig. 8.12). Meningoencephaloceles contain neurons and neuropil, which is a fine fibrillar eosinophilic extracellular material (Figs. 8.13a, b, 8.14, and 8.15).

Differential Diagnosis

If the meningothelial (or neuroglial) nature of the proliferation is recognized, the diagnosis is relatively straightforward. Initial evaluation of meningoceles with a prominent cystic of pseudovascular pattern may raise consideration of vascular neoplasms like hemangioma or angiosarcoma. For additional considerations see "Cutaneous meningioma."

Additional Reading

Cutaneous Meningioma

Argenyi ZB, Thieberg MD, Hayes CM, Whitaker DC. Primary cutaneous meningioma associated with von Recklinghausen's disease. J Cutan Pathol. 1994;21(6):549–56.

Barr RJ, Yi ES, Jensen JL, Wuerker RB, Liao SY. Meningioma-like tumor of the skin. An ultrastructural and immunohistochemical study. Am J Surg Pathol. 1993;17(8):779–87.

Appendix: Practical Approach to Neural Tumors – Flowcharts and Differential Diagnostic Tables

Table A.1 Classification of cutaneous neural tumors

- **Cutaneous peripheral nerve sheath proliferations**
  - Hamartomas
    - True neuromas
      - Palisaded encapsulated neuroma/solitary circumscribed neuroma
      - Mucosal neuroma
  - Fibrolipomatous hamartoma of nerve
  - Other nonneoplastic and hyperplastic proliferations
    - Traumatic neuroma
    - Reparative perineurial hyperplasia
    - Morton's neuroma (interdigital neuritis)
    - Epithelial sheath neuroma[a]
  - Benign neoplasms
    - Neurofibroma[a]
    - Schwannoma
    - Granular cell tumor
    - Nerve sheath myxoma
    - Perineurioma
    - Lipoblastic nerve sheath tumor[a]
  - Malignant neoplasms
    - Malignant peripheral nerve sheath tumor
    - Malignant granular cell tumor
- **Cutaneous proliferations of putative neural origin/differentiation**
  - Benign neoplasms
    - Neurothekeoma
  - Malignant neoplasms
    - Primary cutaneous neuroendocrine carcinoma (Merkel cell carcinoma)
  - Neurofollicular hamartoma
- **Cutaneous neuroblastic and ganglionic proliferations**
  - Benign neoplasms
    - Ganglioneuroma
    - Ganglion cell choristoma[a]
  - Malignant neoplasms
    - Neuroblastoma
- **Cutaneous glial and meningothelial proliferations**
  - Heterotopias
    - Glial heterotopia (nasal glioma)
    - Meningothelial heterotopia/meningocele
  - Benign neoplasms
    - Cutaneous meningioma

[a]The etiologic nature of these entities is disputed or not decidedly established. Neurofibroma is included under the neoplastic group for historical purposes

Z. Argenyi and C.H. Jokinen (eds.), *Cutaneous Neural Neoplasms*, Current Clinical Pathology, DOI 10.1007/978-1-60327-582-8, © Springer Science+Business Media, LLC 2011

Table A.2 Main immunohistochemical findings of common cutaneous neural neoplasms

Marker	S-100	Coll IV	NF	NSE	CD57 (Leu-7)	MBP	GFAP	EMA	VIM	SY	CD34	Other/miscellaneous
Tumor												
Neurofibroma	++	++	+	++	+/–	+/–	–/+	–/+	++	–	++	
Schwannoma	+++	+++	–*	++	++	++	–/+	+capsule	++	–	+/–	
Traumatic neuroma	+++	+++	+++	++	++	++	–	++	++	–	+	
PEN	+++	+++	+++	++	++	++	–	+capsule	++	–	+	
Nerve sheath myxoma	+	+	–	–/+	+/–	–/+	–	+capsule	++	–	–/+	
Cellular neurothekeoma	–	–/+	–	–/+	–/+	–	–	–	++	–	–/+	SMSA, NC1/3
Perineurioma	–	+/–	–	–	–	–	–	+	+	–	+/–	
Granular cell tumor	++	+	–	+	+	+	–	–	++	–	–	CD68, lysozyme
MPNST	+/–	+/–	+/–	+/–	+/–	+/–	–	–	++	–	–/+	Desmin
Nasal glioma	+	+/–	+/–	+	–/+	–/+	+++	–	++	+	–	
Cutaneous meningioma	–/+	–/+	–	–/+	–	–	–	++	+	–	NA	
PNET	–/+	–	–	+	+/–	+/–	–	–	+/–	+	–**	CD99, MB-2
Ganglioneuroma	+	+	+/–	+	+/–	+/–	+/–	–	+	+	NA	
Cutaneous neuroblastoma	–/+	–	–/+	+	+/–	+/–	–	–	+/–	+	**	
PNECS	–	–	+	+	–	–	–	+	–	+/–	–	LMWK, CHG

PEN palisaded encamsulated neuroma, *MPNST* malignant peripheral nerve sheath tumor, *PNET* peripheral neuroectodermal tumor, *PNECS* neuroendocrine carcinoma of the skin, *S-100* S-100 protein, *Coll IV* collagen type IV, *NF* neural filaments, *NSE* neuron-specific enolase, *MPB* myelin basic protein, *GFAP* glial fibrillary acidic protein, *EMA* epithelial membrane antigen, *VIM* vimentin, *SY* synaptophysin, *CD99* antibody to p30/32 mic2, *MB-2* antibody to B-cell lymphoid determinations, *LMWK* low molecular weight keratin, *CHR* chromogranin, *NC1/3* melanoma marker, + weak or focal immunoreactivity, ++ fairly consistent reactivity, +++ usually strong immunoreactivity, +/– variable, immunoreactivity often present, –/+ variable, immunoreactivity often absent, – negative immunoreactivity, *NA* not applicable, * reaction only at nerve of origin, ** only a few cases studied

Table A.3 Histologic differential diagnostic features of cutaneous neoplasms with plexiform growth

	PPEN	PNF	PS	CNSM	PFHT	PSCN
Location in the skin	Superficial dermis	Deep dermis or subcutis	Superficial or deep dermis	Superficial or deep dermis	Deep dermis or subcutis	Mid or upper dermis
Growth pattern	Plexiform or multinodular	Plexiform	Plexiform and multinodular	Lobulated or plexiform	Plexiform and multinodular	Plexiform fascicles in wedge-shape
Encapsulation	Yes, superficially incomplete	Yes, superficially incomplete	Yes	Yes, superficially incomplete	None	None
Constituent cell types	Uniform spindle cells (Schwann cells)	Spindle cells: Schwann cells Perineurial cells Fibroblasts	Spindle cells (Schwann cells)	Spindle and stellate cells Giant cells	Fibroblasts Histiocytic cells Giant cells	Spindle cells, some with mucin
Cytologic pleomorphism	None	None (if present may indicate malignancy)	Often	Rarely	Rarely	Mild
Mitotic figures	None	None	None to rare, but not abnormal	None to rare	None to rare	Rare
Nuclear palisading	Yes, variable	None to rare	Frequent	None	None	None
Verocay bodies	Rare	None	Frequent	None	None	None
Nerve fibers	Usually abundant	Rare, scattered	None	None	None	None
Other features	Focal fibrosis and mucin increase	Focally increased mucin or fibrosis	Predominantly hypercellular	Lymphocytes, abundant mucin	Lymphocytes Microhemorrhages	Periadnexal, perineurial spread

PPEN plexiform, palisaded, encapsulated neuroma, *PNF* plexiform neurofibroma, *PS* plexiform schwannoma, *CNSM* classical nerve sheath myxoma, *PFHT* plexiform fibrohistiocytic tumor, *PSCN* plexiform spindle cell nevus

Adapted with permission from Argenyi ZB. Recent developments in cutaneous neural neoplasms. J Cutan Pathol. 1993;20:97–108

Table A.4 Immunohistochemical reactivity of small round cell cutaneous tumors

	S-100	CK	CEA	EMA	LCA	VIM	CHG	SYN	Leu-7	DES	AC	NSE	NF	CD99
PNECS (Merkel cell tumor)	–	+	–	+	–	–	+	–	–	–	–	+	+/–	–
PNET (neuroblastoma)	–	–	–	–	–	+	+/–	+/–	+/–	–	–	–	+/–	+
Malignant lymphoma	–	–	–	–	+	+	–	–	–	–	–	–	–	+/–
Poorly differentiated eccrine carcinoma	+/–	+	+	+	–	–	–	–	–	–	–	–	–	–
Small cell melanoma	+	–	–	–	–	+	–	–	–	–	–	+	–	–
Embryonal rhabdomyosarcoma	+/–	–	–	–	–	+	–	–	–	+	+	–	–	–

PNECS primary neuroendocrine carcinoma of the skin, *PNET* peripheral neuroectodermal tumor, *NF* neural filaments, *AC* actin, *S-100* S-100 protein, *CK* cytokeratin, *CEA* carcinoembryonic antigen, *EMA* epithelial membrane antigen, *LCA* leukocyte common antigen, *VIM* fimentin, *CHG* chromograninm, *SYN* synaptophysin, *DES* desmin, *NSE* neuron specific enolase, *CD99* antibody to p 30/32, *CD99 may not be expressed in primary mature neuroblastomas, + present, – absent, +/– variable present

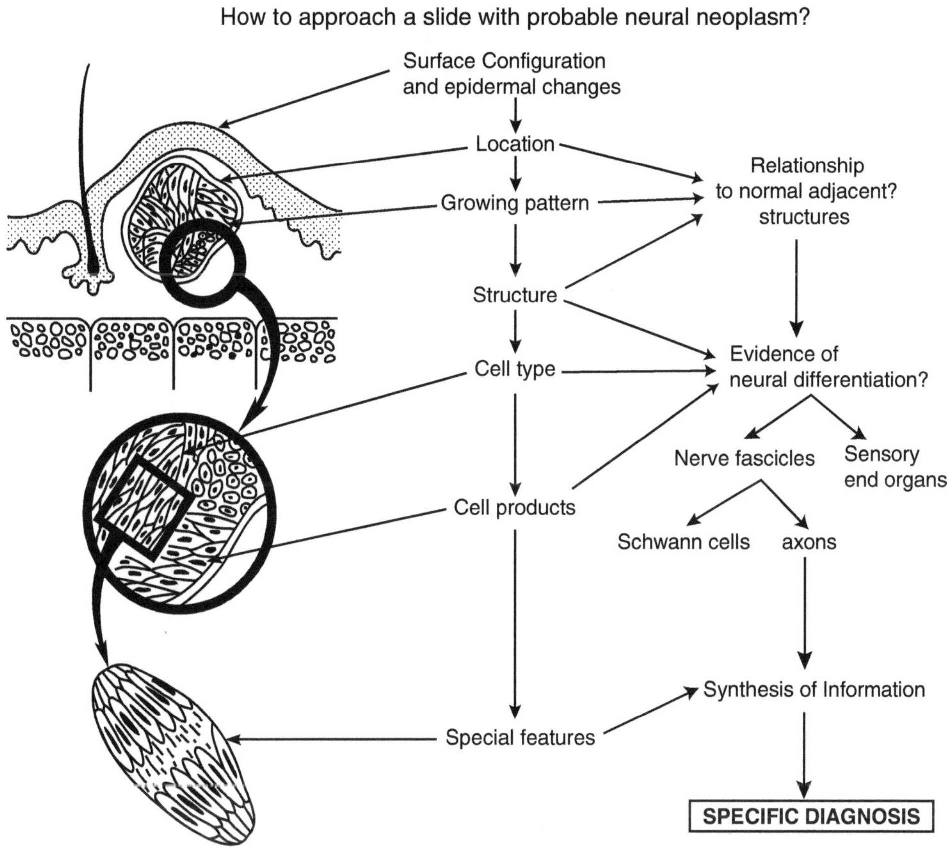

Fig. A.1 How to approach a slide with probable neural neoplasm? (artwork by ZA)

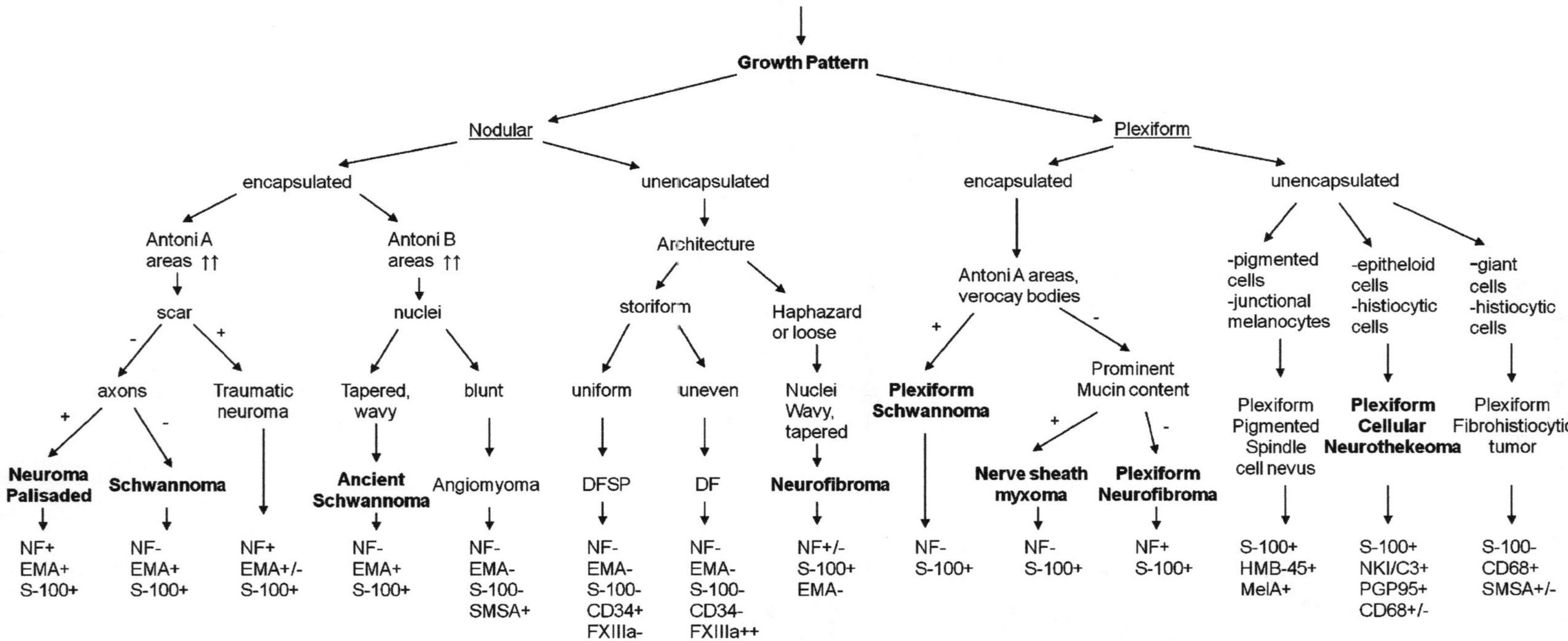

Abbreviations: DF: dermatofibroma, DFSP: dermatofibrosarcoma protuberans, EMA: epithelial membran antigen, NF: neuralfilament, S-100 S-100 Protein, SMSA: smooth muscle specified actin, MelA, PGP95: protein gene product

Fig. A.2 An algorithmic approach of the diagnosis of common cutaneous neural neoplasms (artwork by ZA)

Index

P

MIX
Papier aus verantwortungsvollen Quellen
Paper from responsible sources
FSC® C105338

If you have any concerns about our products,
you can contact us on
ProductSafety@springernature.com

In case Publisher is established outside the EU,
the EU authorized representative is:
Springer Nature Customer Service Center GmbH
Europaplatz 3, 69115 Heidelberg, Germany

Printed by Libri Plureos GmbH
in Hamburg, Germany